"Debbie Potts depicts her j[ourney through] multiple health setbacks. [She has developed the] Wholestic Method that will [improve your health,] happiness, and prosperity. [...] anecdotal information that Debbie shares so eloquently. [...] book and your life will be better. *Life is Not a Race... it is a Journey* is a **must read** and her The WHOLESTIC Method is a **must follow**. Read it now... Thank me later!"

Todd Durkin, MA, CSCS
Owner, Fitness Quest 10
Lead Training Advisor, Under Armour
Author, The WOW BOOK

"Debbie's story and solution will change your WHOLE life. The deep, breadth, and sincerity of Debbie's journey is as instructional as it is inspirational. Feeling better, working better, performing better, and living your best is possible. Debbie will tell you how. Stop your racing! Read and live this book."

Larry Indiviglia
Fitness Professional, Coach, and Author

"*Life is not a Race* is an incredibly important book for these chaotic times. There is a "busy" epidemic everywhere I look. Empty nesters who have raised four children are so busy and stressed even though their kids are out of the house and they did not go back to work. What is happening in our society? This busy epidemic can become dangerous when the Type A athlete pushes themselves to the limit, causing sometimes irreparable damage to their cardiovascular systems and HPA axis. Debbie bares all as she shares her story of becoming one of the top triathletes to experiencing crippling health issues and then her long road to recovery. She has created The WHOLESTIC Method to help people who are already burned out and others to prevent this burnout. This information is critical for anyone who has the business disease."

Ronda Collier
CEO and Co-Founder
SweetWater Health, LLC
www.BeatHealthy.com

"Debbie's dedication to being on the forefront of the science of exercise makes all the difference in the results of training with her. In this book, Debbie humbly shares the deeply personal health journey she has been on, all that she knew before was completely turned upside down, and what she found has made her healthier than the nationally rated triathlete she was before it happened to her!"

Sarah Hasselbeck
Athlete and Coach

"Debbie Potts delivers a very valuable and thoughtful message that is enriched by her personal experience of reaching great athletic heights and suffering from serious health setbacks. Her The WHOLESTIC method can benefit endurance athletes trying to balance challenging workouts with a busy, stressful modern life. For the highly motivated, goal-oriented, Type-A mindset that is so common in the endurance scene, Debbie's message can be life changing. There is plenty of cookie cutter training advice out there of limited value, but Debbie's book will have deep and lasting significance for how you approach the sport and make sensible training decisions that benefit your long-term progress and also protect your health."

Brad Kearns
Former national champion and #3 world-ranked professional triathlete
co-author of Primal Endurance, host of Primal Endurance Podcast

"The accumulation of stress, in all its forms—physical, biochemical and mental-emotional—is a primary cause of most health and fitness problems. Even when eating right and exercising well, excess stress can disrupt our best-laid plans. Debbie's book can help guide us out of the rat race and onto a better journey."

Dr. Phil Maffetone
author, clinician, and researcher

"Brilliantly said, Debbie! I applaud you for sharing your story and helping others to realize that being a "human doing" instead of a "human being" is a recipe for disaster. It takes courage to buck our cultural norms of being rewarded for over-achieving at the cost of all else. Thank you for giving others permission to truly listen to their bodies so they not only survive but thrive."

Dr. Amanda Brimhall
Naturopathic Physician and Functional Medicine Practitioner

"Potts chronicles her own journey from driven to breakdown to reinvention. The first two parts are where Debbie learned what didn't work in terms of life health. It's the third part that is what makes this book so valuable! Dive in. See where you might be on this journey. Use the principles that Potts shares to make a true assessment of your life and your health. Create your own personal story of what real success means."

Mark Allen
6-Time Hawaii IRONMAN World Champion
http://markallencoaching.com

"This is an important book to read for all of us who tend to overdo life. Overtraining, overeating, overworking have become hallmarks of modern life. Our stress response has its limits. *Life Is Not a Race* will help you identify your state of stress and how you can begin to reset yourself back to a state of balance."

Dr. Dan Kalish
Founder, The Kalish Institute

"As a physician, I see a spectrum of patients: some are sick because of unhealthy lifestyle choices, but a surprising number are unwell despite doing everything right. The conventional biomedical world has slowly been catching up to the scientific benefits of optimal living, but people need answers for what to do right now, every day. Debbie takes us on her personal journey through the murky weeds that comprise the current frontiers of health. She makes a compelling argument for toxicities inherent to our modern lifestyle and defines a clear road map towards wellness and balance.

Emily Y. Wong, MD, MHA, FACP, LMCHK
Affiliate Associate Professor, University of Washington
http://imi.com.hk/dr-emily-y-wong-general-practitioner-hong-kong.html

"Over the past ten years, I have learned important lessons from Debbie as client seeing her once a week for personal training and coaching. Now Debbie is encouraging all of us to take our learning to the next level by understanding the real costs of our lifestyle and the constant drive and desire to do more. For Type A individuals, this book will force you to pause and think about the impact of your life. What is really important to you and why? Debbie forces her readers to think about the ramifications of their lifestyle choices and shares her very personal lessons – a gift. How many of us take pride in squeezing every drop of life out of every minute of every day. Debbie shares important lessons for all of us about the flip side of living large."

Clayton Lewis
Arivale CEO and Co-founder
Your Scientific Path to Wellness

LIFE IS NOT A RACE...
IT IS A JOURNEY

Learn how to pace the WHOLE you with The WHOLESTIC Method

by Debbie Potts

Copyright© 2016 Debbie Potts
Life is Not a Race... It Is a Journey
All rights reserved.
ISBN-10: 1540572005
ISBN-13: 978-1540572004

Published by Cardinal Rules Press
Cover design by uk.fiverr.com/nisha
Edited and formatted by Marley Gibson

Although the author and publisher have made every effort to ensure the information in this book was correct at press time, the author and publisher do not assume and hereby disclaim any liability to any party for any loss, damage, or disruption caused by errors or omissions, whether such errors or omissions result from negligence, accident, or any other cause.

This publication is intended to provide helpful and informative material. It is not intended to diagnose, treat, cure, or prevent any health problem or condition, nor is it intended to replace the advice of a physician. No action should be taken solely on the contents of this book. The anecdotes and advice in this book are not intended as a substitute for the medical advice of physicians or health care professionals. Always consult your physician or qualified healthcare professional on any matters regarding your health and before adopting any suggestions in this book or drawing inferences from it.

Any and all product names referenced within this book are the trademarks of their respective owners. None of these owners have sponsored, authorized, endorsed, or approved this book. Always read all information provided by the manufacturers' product labels before using their products. The author and publisher are not responsible for claims made by manufacturers.

Printed in the United States.

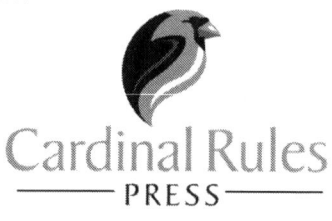

Contents

Foreword 1
Prologue -A Word from the Author 5
1 The Fall from the Peak of the Mountain Top 21
2 Burnout, Blow up, and Breakdown 33
3 The Thrill of Victory 51
4 The Bus Ride that Changed my World 77
5 Everything Happens for a Reason 99
6 Running from a Lion 113
7 What is Adrenal Dysfunction? 125
8 Your Greatest Wealth is Health 133
9 Giving Your Body a Tune Up 151
10 To Burn Sugar or to Burn Fat? That is the Question 167
11 Elements of The WHOLESTIC Method 181
12 The Pursuit of Happiness 187
13 A Rehab Center for Busy-ness Addiction? 205
14 The World of Podcasting 209
15 A Reflection on my Healing Journey 215
16 The Attempt to Return to Racing 235
17 That was then… This is now 251
18 The Butterfly Transformation into the WHOLE Person 263
19 Chasing the Dream 267
20 To Pace or to Race in Life? 271
Epilogue - The WHOLE Transformation Ongoing Process 279
About the Author 283

Foreword

I once told Debbie Potts I had to pass on a bike workout. You see, Debbie is always trying to include people; in a workout, a trail run, or a track workout.

She was coaching and training a triathlete who was preparing for his second Ironman event. They were getting on their bikes when she asked me if I wanted to join them for an hour. I knew how hard they would train and I said lightly, "I won't be able to keep up." As I was walking away to take lunch, she shouted out with a surprised tone, "But, we're on stationary bikes!"

It's not often you come across a woman as motivated as Debbie Potts. You have to be motivated to complete fifteen Ironman events and I don't even know how many marathons. She is a businesswoman, a coach, a trainer, and an accomplished athlete. She is one of the most committed and generous trainers I have come across. She is always willing to introduce, connect, and include. I knew her when she was back from her Kona Ironman World Championships in 2012 and I knew her when she started hitting the wall of fatigue and training burnout only a few months later.

In my career as a soft tissue and sports therapist, I have worked with a large number of endurance athletes. Some people think they are absolutely nuts. After all, who likes to run for fifty kilometers or to throw in a marathon set after a long bike ride? To me, endurance athletes hone and polish a mindset that is essential for serious athletes. There is a clear desire for measured progress.

I saw this mindset working in Dave Scott and his athletes in Colorado. I started working with a lot of triathletes early on in my career because I liked how motivated they were. With my background in martial arts, I was familiar with the tedium of practicing something over and over again. In the swim, bike, and run, triathletes understand small changes lead to big gains over time.

People who log twenty hours a week of training take their time seriously. Working with Debbie reminded me a lot of the Olympians I worked with at the Olympic Training Center in California. It takes a certain conviction to be a career athlete with a deep commitment to detail and consistency. There is also a constant search for new techniques and strategies to get more out of training.

Maintaining such a high training load can carry a lot of hidden costs. As much as we live in a culture that likes to track progress, we don't always pay attention to the resources being drained. When Debbie came back from racing Kona that year, she had that deep Hawai'i tan, a personal glow of doing well and the satisfaction of supporting her clients and friends. She was in her element.

She logged her hours, stayed consistent, and achieved so much. Yet, within a few months, she told me her legs were on fire from short workouts, she was tired all the time, and she had to pull out of races.

What had changed so much in such a small window of time? How did a top athlete go from an eight-minute mile for the length of a marathon at the end of an Ironman to a ten-minute mile on short runs that left her with unexplainable fatigue?

Life is Not a Race is about adrenal dysfunction from the perspective of an accomplished endurance athlete and a dedicated trainer. Debbie wasn't willing to quit her athletic life despite being held back by a chronically poor recovery and with very little help from conventional medicine. Debbie had to reach out to expert after expert in the field of health because she was dealing with an issue that is under-reported and under-researched.

Adrenal dysfunction falls within a category of illness that is poorly managed by modern medicine. So much in fact that there are still doctors who refuse to accept it as a diagnosis. The standard tests used in conventional medicine are too wide to properly analyze cortisol and hormone levels and are unable to identify this serious issue. Many people go undiagnosed and suffer daily because of it.

While medicine has come a long way since the 1980s when most of society would discount notions of Lyme's Disease, Hypothyroidism, and Fibromyalgia with the phrase, "It's all in your head," we are still far from understanding all the disease patterns afflicting us. When conventional labs fail to lead to a specific diagnosis, you may need to start exploring other options and find experts and doctors willing to advocate for your health.

That is what Debbie did. Her story, *Life is Not a Race*, is a critical guide for athletes and non-athletes alike. She found a way to regain her health and develop a method that helps others. She dug deeply into a modern epidemic and she has come out the other side with a message that is loud and clear: **We don't have to suffer from adrenal dysfunction. We don't have to live every day as a race. We need to be the best advocates for our own health.**

Read this book. Think about what red flags and stressors are holding you back. Think about what you can change in your daily routine to better cultivate your health. And, know when you work with the right knowledge, you can achieve phenomenal things.

Scott Olsen
Soft Tissue Therapist, Movement Coach, and Qigong Teacher
San Diego, CA
www.beyondthemuscle.com

Prologue
A Word from the Author

"Life is like the ocean. It can be calm, or still and rough or ridged, but in the end, it is always beautiful."
- Unknown

In the spring of 2013, I went on a long bike ride—typical of any other weekend—with my husband, Neal, and one of our training partners. However, instead of getting a spirited and satisfying workout, I found myself crumpled over on the side of the road in tears.

I was weak and lethargic. My legs would not keep pedaling or working anymore. I pulled over to the shoulder and had the first of what would soon be many meltdowns.

At the time, I was a top age group strong triathlete who often placed top on the bike segment in a triathlon with a reputation of competing in races around the area, as well as in the annual Hawaii World Championships. A few months prior to my roadside debacle, I was in peak racing shape—lean, strong, and powerful—finishing my best triathlon season in twelve years.

Who would have ever predicted I would suddenly be overpowered with fatigue and emotions on the side of the road - especially on my bike of all things.

That day, not only was I unable to continue the bike ride, but soon began to quickly gain weight and lose muscle mass. My body was changing on the outside even though I thought I was eating right with a real food diet full of healthy fats, moderate proteins, and low carbohydrates and doing all the right types of exercises for triathlon training.

I was "Debbie Diesel" and the picture of health to everyone around me. What was going on inside my body that forced me to crawl back onto my bike just to make it home? Also, I wasn't fitting into my clothes, I was getting headaches from certain foods, and I was feeling depressed and impatient.

This wasn't me. This didn't resemble anything even in the neighborhood of me.

I loved owning my own fitness studio, enjoyed working with my clients, as well as training and racing in triathlons. I thought I was doing things for my health to help me become stronger, fitter, leaner, and faster while having fun, smiling, and laughing. I needed immediate answers and results to explain what was going on with me. I was on a mission to figure out why I couldn't train, sleep, or lose weight. I mean, I had goals, race plans, and scheduled commitments the rest of 2013. I didn't have time for setbacks.

But, I was in for the biggest impediment of all.

How much can we push the envelope without exploding, burning out, and breaking down? I liked to push myself and I lived with the mentality that "more is better" if I was going to be successful in all areas of life. Perfectionist? Possibly. Type A Personality? Yeah, sure. I'll admit I'm perhaps "Type A" personality with a little ADD thrown in. I thrive on being busy and feel as if I am wasting time if I am not doing something.

I am sure you can relate to this addiction of being busy as well as having a monkey brain mentality. Most of us are unable to focus on one task at a time or shut off our mind, especially when trying to sleep at night. Not me.

Every minute of the day, we demand our body to respond and adjust to our excessive busyness or various sources of stressors. Our body doesn't know the difference between stress from a severe infection or even a death in the family to eating a poor diet or over-scheduling ourselves day after day. We literally overload ourselves with some type of stress from multiple sources. Then, one day, the body says no more and you can no longer respond to the stressful source, toxin, event, or situation.

Stress is stress. We all have a different capacity to tolerate various loads and levels of it. Each individual's capacity to respond to stress also varies over time per one of the experts, Dr. James Wilson, author of the "Adrenal Fatigue: The 21st Century Stress Syndrome."

You may not do triathlons, marathons, or do cycling events, but you may work full time while balancing a family life, or you have lifestyle habits that include energy "robbers" and living in a toxic environment. People, work, home, environment and the food we eat can all be sources of stress, or rather "energy robbers," as Dr. Wilson explains in his book.

How do we stop this horrendous cycle we've gotten ourselves into? We've got to put more speed bumps in our day and learn how to quiet our minds. What are we teaching our children and our society?

Doing more is not the answer. Speeding is not allowed on certain streets or the highway – and we have speed limits to follow by law or else we are fined or hopefully just a warning. Should we not set some speed limits in life?

As you will learn from my experience—and do take notes so you don't experience what I have since 2013—speeding through each day and every activity is not the road to success. We need to find a detour when we finally get a roadblock in the path, forcing us to take an alternative direction in life. Life is not to be a race to the finish line, especially if the finish line is not only your bed at night, rather you are driving yourself to another "bed" – your death bed if you continue. Don't do what I've done when my life became a constant race without any recovery time for so many years that I had no idea it was not good for me- just the opposite. I thought I was doing the "right" thing to be a healthy and fit individual.

My life felt happy, satisfying, and rewarding. I loved what I was doing and I had no regrets. But, as you will learn more about my experience, too much of anything can become toxic and too little of anything can create deficiencies.

Stressors don't have to feel like stress as we know it, like yelling and screaming at someone. Stress on our body is sneaky and hidden until one day we finally are forced to listen to our body calling for help and attention from the inside out. My bike ride experiencing in early spring of 2013 was the beginning of my body crying for attention.

Focus people… focus.

Are you constantly on the go?

Are you a slave to your "to-do" list and feel like you don't have enough hours in the day to make it all happen?

Do you find yourself obsessively checking your cell phone multiple times throughout the day?

I'm guilty of all the above. Especially the attachment to my phone. I check it way too much and it drives me crazy. Why do I have to see who liked my post on Instagram or who texted me? What was that notification for? And, whose call did I miss?

I mean, I need to check my messages for work as I own my business and train clients every weekday. I don't want to shirk my duties or make people think I'm not interested in them.

But, the thing is, I find focusing on doing one thing at a time and being set in the here and now is a major challenge. The end result is multitasking, trying to do everything at once, and being distracted.

In this day and age with so many responsibilities, so much involvement, and the hurriedness of trying to balance work and home life, we are always dealing with a project or talking to someone, managing this, that, or the other, but at the same time, we are wondering what we are doing right after that or if we should be somewhere else at same time. Some people call this" FOMO" or Fear of Missing Out.

How many times do *you* check your email or messages each day and this hit "refresh" a minute later to see if you missed anything? Do you have FOMO?

More and more, I am observing how mentally scattered and disconnected we are with ourselves. In the twenty-five years I have been a personal fitness trainer, as well my eight years as a fitness studio owner, too many people walk in exhausted, flustered, distracted, and anxious as if they're in a marathon.

Why are we running from a lion all day long and living life as a race? We are just completing one meeting or appointment and then our mind jumps ahead to focus on where we are heading next or who we are meeting with or who's picking the kids up, and, God forbid, what's for dinner?

This is no way to live, but this has become an acceptable—and expected—way to operate daily in our society. More is better mentality and the glorification of being busy. Are we really busy or just wasting too much time trying to feel or look busy? We begin to be disconnected to our own self and losing our awareness to be in touch with what we feel, see and experience.

When a new client comes into my studio, I usually start them out with a new client posture and movement assessment. In our first session, I get to know their mindset with their health history, relationship with food, their digestion, daily movement patterns, injuries, exercise habits, sleep, stress and more. This information is a crucial first step of what I call The WHOLESTIC Method approach. In our first exercise session, I have the client perform a push, pull, rotation, plank, and a squat movement in order to evaluate their new "natural" movement patterns. From my experience, what surprises me is how often clients are disconnected with their own body.

Many of us find it challenging to learn how to stabilize, isolate, or engage our muscles because we have become so detached from our mind-body connection. We have an inability to focus on ourselves and to quiet the mind and listen to what our body is telling us.

New clients typically struggle with understanding how to feel a muscle activated or how to hold a proper "athletic stance" squat position correctly. Why do so many people find it challenging to stabilizing their shoulders or hold a neutral pelvis while moving their arms or spine? Do we not have self-body awareness anymore? *Or* is it because we don't know how to focus on one thing- including what we feel from the inside out. Rather, most of us are too distracted with other "priorities" on our "to-do" lists in our head that we can't concentrate on other the present. We are always thinking in the past or in the future... but what about being in the present? If we can't activate our glutes (booty), brace our core, anchor our feet into the ground, or have awareness of where our body is in space when we exercise, then how are we able to catch the red flags of chronic stress from living daily life?

What about you?

Do we need to post sticky notes around our home or office to remind us to focus, not get sidetracked and, instead, be more present in the here and now? How many reminders do we need to post on the bathroom mirror and the fridge to set speed limits in daily life? How can we remember to slow down, drink water, move more, and breathe slowly? One way to take care of ourselves is to love who we are and to be more grateful and appreciative of what we do have in our life rather than focus on what we don't have. I suggest that we make "wellness deposits" each day and make an effort to take less "withdrawals."

I like to think of your personal "Wellness Bank Account" where you set goals to create a higher balance in your personal "wellness wealth." If we could only make more positive "Wellness" deposits each day by doing more positive things for ourselves. Instead, most of us automatically give more to others and focus on everyone else but ourselves. As the flight attendant tells us on every journey: "Put your oxygen mask on first before assisting others with theirs." Are we able to make more deposits for ourselves to avoid a negative balance in our personal "wellness bank account?"

Examples of the things I suggest to my clients of The WHOLESTIC Method include:

- Writing in a *Gratitude Journal* each day about what was a positive experience or what you were grateful for that day.
- Taking a walk outside without looking at the phone or listening to music. Just be present with what you are seeing, feeling, and breathing.

- Take five minutes to lie down and do breathing exercises.
- Go get a foot massage or pedicure by yourself and just be still (no phone).
- When in your car in traffic, turn off the news and listen to relaxing, calming or happy music.
- Turn off the TV at home and go outside for a walk. Breathe in fresh air and look at the trees, birds, and sky.
- Walk in your bare feet in your backyard and get connected to the outdoors – and what you feel.

I firmly believe we are creating our own chronic stress by mastering the "art of busy-ness." We spend way too much time being available and connecting with everyone else except ourselves. And, because of this, we keep pushing and pushing, going full steam until our engine blows up. How many times a day do you hit "refresh" button on your email or social media pages? We live each day as we are playing slot machines. We have lost the ability to disconnect, slow down, and relax.

Like the title, *Life is Not a Race*, says, I think about how fast we pace ourselves through the day and I have started to wonder if we need to set speed limits on life? We often put our days on "cruise control" and adjust it off when we hit the pillow at night (and hopefully fall asleep.)

We are designed to vary our speed each day… speed up then slow down, rest then go again. Instead, we are trying to change our engine to be one speed only: fast-paced life speed. We can't override the way we are designed as humans. We need to live life at a variable pace. Perhaps we have to learn the hard way—as I did—once we are put out of commission. It's then we learn the lesson to pace ourselves through life.

My story about living my daily life as a race has nothing to do with participating in Ironman Triathlons, rather it's about how we are adding too much to our daily schedules that can lead to overload on the mind and body—or what I am now calling "chronic stress disease." You could be a single parent of three kids working full time or you could be a CEO of a major company with high expectations. Whatever "busy-ness" is saturating your day, it is all the same. Too much of anything can lead to toxicity. We are accumulating too much stress. We can only tolerate so much before we combust internally.

I should know, because not only did my life blow up, my entire bodily train derailed.

I have a long-time client who is a busy, successful CEO who has started up of many top companies. His specialty is managing his teams and keeping them productive by encouraging them to FOCUS on their business goals, assignments or projects due. If we could learn how to *focus* on one thing right now then we might not get distracted (*Look... squirrel!*) and we could complete the task at hand and then move on to the next item on our to-do list. I am discovering a common challenge in today's society. My "area of opportunity" is the ability to *focus* on one thing. The word *focus* has been my theme word the in past years for my business. Then, the keyword became *transformation*, and now I use the phrase "**Live from the inside out**." You will soon find out why.

Life is Not a Race chronicles my journey from being a top female triathlete to a stressed out woman with adrenal dysfunction. I was sidelined and am still repairing from the damage, with a domino effect of hormonal imbalances and more. From my experience with adrenal dysfunction, I started a mission to find a new journey to improve the WHOLE me from the inside out in order to heal and recover my health. In the process, I created The WHOLESTIC Method, an evolutionary way to transform the WHOLE body and mind our performance in life and sports from the inside out. We will touch upon my "Red Flags" and eight of the elements of The WHOLESTIC Method that focus on improving our resiliency to daily life in order to improve fat loss, health, and performance.

What in the world am I talking about? Most people don't understand what I'm talking about when I say adrenal dysfunction. Most still don't know until now… until I share my story.

The point of this book is not to explain how the brain, HPA Axis, hormonal, and body systems work; that is not my expertise (check out my resource page). My mission in writing this book is to help you transform the WHOLE you with The WHOLESTIC Method—based on my experience in order to avoid getting to the stage of exhaustion I experienced.

Throughout my story, I will use the term adrenal dysfunction to simplify the discussion, but the word "HPA Axis" is used more often as new research is discovered, as I've said. I will dive into my experience of this internal crash of my body systems and trying to learn the root cause that activates the domino effect in the body.

While my story is from an endurance athlete's perspective on life, athletes of all levels can benefit from the lessons learned in my journey. I believe most all of us are too busy, too distracted, and too scheduled every day. I have learned that stress comes in different forms. You may not feel stressed, (the brain stops noticing anything familiar even if it is dysfunctional), but you are creating stress in your body that your brain will interpret as a threat and; therefore, release stress hormones.

We could all benefit from learning how to improve our focus, how to be more present, and be aware of our emotions or what we feel at the moment. We've got to start paying attention to what we are feeling from the inside out. If we could focus on what we feel physically, mentally, and emotionally, maybe we begin to grow and transform into a healthier version of ourselves.

Too much of anything is toxic; especially stress, which will influence the whole you and impact:

- your ability to make the best decisions on your food choices
- impact your motivation and ability to exercise
- alter your ability sleep through the night
- motivation and energy to move more during the day
- impair digestion, gut health and food sensitivities
- lead to depression and anxiety

> *"I am strong because I've been weak.*
> *I am fearless because I've been afraid.*
> *I am wise because I've been foolish."*
> *- Unknown*

Sometimes, we need to take a left or right turn instead of staying on the same road. It has taken me almost four years to figure that out.

We are taught a certain way of living, eating, or training so that is how it is done. What about thinking outside of the box and exploring unknown territory? We are influenced on how to live by the food giants and government agencies, as well as drug companies. Sometimes, you have to stop and wonder why we are told to do, live, or eat a certain way. When guidelines, rule, and claims do not make sense to me, I gradually start to challenge the theories of mainstream media.

I didn't understand why we, endurance athletes, were told to consume so many grams of carbohydrates and/or sugar per hour when training and racing. I didn't understand why we were supposed to eat first thing in the morning and then eat small meals throughout the day to keep our metabolism elevated. I didn't understand the guidelines given to diabetics, those with heart disease, and cancer patients from the governing bodies setting the rules. We can't always believe everything we are told, even from our trusted doctor or government agencies. We need to take our health into our own hands and do what works best for us. We are all different and biochemically unique.

The rate of chronic health diseases and obesity are on the rise. Why? Because our nutritional habits and way of living need to be reassessed. We must make a connection between our daily routines and the symptoms we suffer from such as blood sugar imbalances, hormone issues, migraines, asthma, allergies, autism, ADHD, heart disease, etc. We've got to improve our quality of life by working on our nutrition, eating real food (reduce sugar and grains), exercising right, sleeping more, drinking more water, and the focus of my story… to manage our daily stressors.

Based on my observations of clients, friends, and family members, I started to do my own investigation into other methods of how we can all achieve optimal wellness. Our nutritional habits or rather the Standard American Diet (S.A.D.) is an area I hope to specialize in as you will discover more in my The WHOLESTIC Method manual and program. I want to help society improve our eating habits if we want to be healthy by eating real whole foods and eliminating processed foods like sugar and grains.

If I had been able to look into the future, I would have changed a few areas of my daily operation. For some reason, my daily schedule was so packed every single day for **years.** Actually, I thought I was Super Woman, thinking if I could fit more into my day, I'd be tremendously successful. I assumed being busy was a sign of accomplishment. I was organized, scheduled, efficient, and, yes, busy. This was the life and the schedule I knew how to live and, at the time, I was successful at living this way.

Did I feel more successful as a business owner, trainer, coach, and athlete if I packed as much as possible into the day? Perhaps I felt I was being lazy if I sat down to rest or skipped a workout session, or not at work (my fitness studio) all hours of the day. After all, it's what we've been conditioned to think.

Living each day in a constant mode of stress, our adrenaline—or our natural "high on life"—eventually comes crashing down on us from the inside out. We usually are not aware of the warnings or signals until it's too late.

That is, until…

- ✓ You're sore, gaining weight, or haven't had a decent night's sleep in weeks.
- ✓ You're drinking so much coffee and soda that you're twitching and shaking from the caffeinating just to get through the work day and all of your commitments.
- ✓ You're the endorphin high from racing and rushing through the day from sun up to sun down from one activity to the next.

It doesn't matter if you participate in Ironman Triathlons, run a business, work hard for someone else, or fill your day as a stay-at-home parent taking care of the family household. We are too busy and the outcome is not beneficial… until you are forced to push the "pause" and "reset" buttons, as I did.

Ideally, we should wake up feeling energized and ready to face the day with positive enthusiasm, but how many of us are naturally charged up? I see lots of clients every day unknowingly fighting signs of chronic fatigue or adrenal dysfunction and they don't even know it. It just seems to be the norm of living life and being an adult these days. But, it's so much more than that.

So, I share my personal journey which most friends and family members were not aware of. Obviously, the story is emotional to me, as you will find out. After many years, I have finally become aware of my personal red flags or stressor alerts. I was oblivious to the signals my body was sending me at the time. It took years for me to discover that my "normal" way of life was actually harming my health instead of enhancing it, even though I was doing strength training and yoga, as well as swimming, biking, and running. I realized, after the fact, that my internal health breakdown was not only from my exercise training and racing, but how I dealt with daily life.

Through the years, I was forced to transform myself into a new person. In order to pull out of the hole I'd dug myself into (unknowingly, of course), I had to commit to a major life overhaul: my daily habits, work schedule, coaching commitments, and training routine all needed to be re-evaluated. Just as in any emergency situation, I had to become my own first responder and assess the situation in order to heal myself. The lessons we learn in life are not so obvious until we step away and look back at them.

As I write about my experiences, I finally get it. By writing about what I went through, I've had a major "Ah-ha."

moment. I never really stopped being busy before. My attempt to find answers to my problems was only adding another type of stress. By pausing to reflect on the last few years, I understood everything.

We all need to stop living life in the fast lane with the cruise control button on non-stop. We must cut down on our multi-tasking, getting distracted, and instead become more grounded with who we are now. We have to learn how to crawl before we can stand and eventually walk. Now, we have to relearn how to pick ourselves back up, stand up tall, move right and play in daily life. We can't learn new habits if we don't have any awareness that we are broken in the first place. What are you doing, experiencing, or feeling right this moment?

Let's dig deeper into my very personal journey that I share with the hopes that my breakdown will help you connect with yourself and avoid burnout. I want you to learn how to push pause, reset, and re-calibrate your brain (the commander-in-charge) and your body.

I want you to come away from this book with the notion that you need to live your life in the present, not as a daily race.

Keep reading to find out why…

The Fall from the Peak of the Mountain Top

1

"The 3 Cs in Life: 1) Choice, 2) Chance, 3) Change. You must make the choice to take the chance if you want anything in life to change."
- Unknown

You're sound asleep, dreaming of a cerulean blue Hawaiian vacation when all of a sudden... *BEEP, BEEP, BEEP.*

The startling and ear-piercing roar of the alarm clock jolts you out of your peaceful paradise. The intrusion creates an instant chaos inside your mind and body. Your heart rate increases, your adrenalin begins to flow like the automatic drip from the brewing coffee, and your instinctual "fight or flight" kicks in activating your nervous system to scream out at you to "Get moving. Get up now or you will be attacked." It is time to run from a lion... your first "interval training session" of the day.

Your start line may not be the deep water start in Kona, but it may be jumping into a cold shower to start your race day. Maybe your day begins by waking up your kids, preparing breakfast for the family or roommates while also taking care of yourself and prepare for your day—showering, dressing, and major multitasking.

Of course, you can't help checking messages, emails, and social media updates at the same time as eating, drinking coffee, and then dressing. We hit cruise control, go all day long until it is over, and then we reach our own finish line – our bed. The day isn't just battling one attack then rest, recover, and repair before the next round, instead, we are continuously fighting the daily battles of life.

This constant demand on our internal emergency response system team (the HPA Axis) wears out the messenger. The continuous mental disarray and lack of focus from our multi-tasking aren't "normal" for our body. Our 'car' is going to eventually break down on the side of the road and someone is going to come help pick you up and send you to the repair shop to get an overhaul. That person is only going to be *you*.

Living this way is not natural. It's frenetic. It's harried. All day long, your body and mind go through your own type of transition of daily life. It may not just be from the swim to the bike to the run, but now we experience different obligations we are required to attend to each day. You may have to take care of others before yourself, including driving your kids to school, then commuting to your workplace, all while battling the traffic, weather, or train delays... not to mention finding a place to park.

You finally reach your workplace only to delve into the first events of the fully-scheduled day and all your "to do" list of responsibilities: reports, meetings, phone calls, customers, and deadlines. You don't slow down until it is time to drive (commute and sit again patiently) home for your next set of events: cooking and serving dinner, family time discussing the day, kids' homework, dishes, laundry, checking email, online activities, getting the kids bathed and into bed, watching television or a movie and maybe spending time with your spouse/significant other before you head to the finish line... bed. You hit the pillow after a long, full day, more than likely completely exhausted, but feeling wired from the stress and bedlam of another race day.

Wow.

Now, take a deep breath in.

That was exhausting just reading about a typical day of a parent working full time.

How do we survive in this race of life?

What is the end result of living each day as a race?

You are wide awake at 2:00 a.m. and your monkey mind won't shut off. Monkey mind is a Buddhist term meaning *"unsettled; restless; capricious; whimsical; fanciful; inconstant; confused; indecisive; uncontrollable."*

This would be me and also many people I observe every day. I am always working in my head on something; my brain is always turned on. I rarely sit and just watch TV or a movie without stretching on the floor, foam roller, or working on my iPad or computer. My mind goes to my "to do" list and adding more to it. Then, I always contemplate what I should be doing and how do I get everything done this week. I need to set priorities or what my business group for fitness professionals does each week (Todd Durkin Mastermind) and create our "BIG FIVE" on Sunday and then meet on an accountability call on Friday to evaluate what we accomplished.

Actually, our stress hormone cortisol is high during the night, making us wired; instead of low while our melatonin is low… the opposite is to happen with our natural circadian rhythm. When we feel sleepy at night (sunset) our melatonin hormone is to rise at the same time our cortisol level dip down. I talk about the hormones cortisol, melatonin, and our natural sleep cycle in my chapter on Sleep in my The WHOLESTIC Method manual. Our constant state of living with stress (remember stress comes from various forms) leaves us wired, but tired. This is all a part of the "red flags" that come from living life as a race and not knowing when to push "pause and reset" to recalibrate the body and the mind. Instead, we end up on a downhill spiral and creating a hormonal imbalance that may take months or years to recover from (at least years for me.)

You stare at the clock, counting the hours until you have to wake up to start another race all over again. You can't stop the clutter in your head. Things like worrying about work, deliberating financial stresses, bills, and payments, or pensive reflections on family issues, the kids' needs, and not spending enough quality time with your spouse. You struggle to fall back asleep and become frustrated and tense rather than relaxing and quieting your mind. Before you know it, the alarm goes off and you can't believe it is morning again.

The race starts again.

Repeat.

It feels like you just finished the previous race and all you want to do is pull the sheets over your face and go back to sleep. We love our precious sleep, but we don't appreciate it enough. Our recovery, rest, and repair time is supposed to occur while we sleep between 10:00 p.m. and 6:00 a.m., but what happens if we are up late at night and then finally fall asleep until around 2:00 a.m. when you are wide awake feeling as if it is time to start your race all over again.

Sleep... we sacrifice our precious slumber in order to do more in the twenty-four hours we have in a day. More is not better, but more sleep may be more important than more busy work.

However, life goes on.

On your mark.

Set.

Go!

Does this sound familiar?

How often do you wake up tired, exhausted, and frazzled? Living life as a race every day puts you in the role of a hamster stuck on a wheel. We wake up tired, overload our bodies with caffeine to keep us awake, supplement it throughout the day, and then, it's no wonder we can't sleep at night because we are wired when it is finally the time to wind down.

We find ourselves in a lather, rinse, repeat habitual behavior.

Our ancestors would be horrified by the schedule we follow day after day that becomes our normal way of living… and expected by others at home and the workplace. We are not designed to live in "fight or flight" mode, rather a balance with "rest and digest." Yin and Yang. Too much or too little of anything is not healthy for anyone from the inside out. We have trained ourselves to not stop until we drop or reach the finish line. Our "normal" way of packing each day to the fullest while always being connected to society and consuming processed sugar filled foods is quickly breaking down our health from the inside out.

What is the result?

We are not designed to run from a lion all day and every day, but that is how society has us wired and expected in order to succeed. When do we stop, pause and be present enough to see the red flags hanging in front of us? Or do we keep on plugging away until we crash and burn?

Maybe this example is familiar to you or you know someone who lives each day this way. We are all in one type of a race or another from the time the alarm (starting gun) goes off in the morning until we hit the pillow and mattress (the finish line).

It is possible you are living life each day as your own race, but you are unaware of the stress you are placing on your body because your race has become the norm for you. Perhaps you are racing to your own "finish line" every day for no specific reason. Just because.

What are we racing toward?

What are we racing from?

What is the purpose of our mission… and why do we put so much pressure on ourselves on a daily basis?

What are we doing to ourselves?

What did I do to myself?

I was at—what I considered to be—the peak of my physical fitness level and triathlon career… and yet, I broke down, crashed and burned from the inside out (not another bike accident or physical injury.). My breakdown was not from getting older… this internal crash in my body became obvious at the age of forty-one which is young in my books.

I went through daily life on cruise control, filling my hours up each day from the time I woke up until I went to bed at night. I sacrificed my sleep at night and my time with my amazing husband to fit more in the day. My pace didn't slow down. There were no rest stops or time to recharge and then go again. The fast paced busy life I lived leads me down the wrong road. My road came to an end… and ran the machine of my internal combustion system out and I became forced to choose a new direction and a new path in life. I crossed the finish line of fifteen Ironman triathlons with success because I paced myself in my training and racing… I built up my aerobic engine the best anyone could possibly do in life and my fat burning capabilities were amazing from the type of metabolic efficiency training. I ate low-carb and healthy fats while avoiding sugar and processed foods. I thought I was doing everything right to improve my health and performance levels to become an elite athlete.

However, I obviously didn't pace myself in my daily life as well as I did on race day.

My health collapsed not only because of my excessive training and racing, but because I was adding this other "part time job" on top of a busy day job with the stress of running my own business, paying an excessive rent each month for my fitness studio, always working on marketing a fitness studio in a competitive market, and then cutting back on sleep to fit it all in every day.

My life was too stressful and as a result of my emergency response system—the adrenal glands—were seemingly overworking for too many years and simply became exhausted. My body and brain became what is known as dysregulated and dysfunctional. My stress hormone, cortisol, was working overtime (higher than normal levels) until I hit exhaustion—now too low of cortisol—as a result of my constant state of being busy.

The hormones that help the brain and body deal with stress (fight or flight system) ended my race schedule to something called adrenal dysfunction (simplified version) that stopped me in my tracks.

We are built to run from a lion quickly and then rest and recover before the next attack happens instead of the life most of us life leads us of running from a metaphorical lion from sunrise to sunset (or longer) without resting and recovering.

Do you also get caught in the high speed of life or do you know how to re-calibrate? I discovered most of us do not see the red flags and respond to the brain-body alerts that we are given over time.

You may enter a whole new world, as I did. As a caterpillar transforms into a new beautiful butterfly, sometimes you must learn how to embrace change and the new you until you transform again in a new better (wiser) version of yourself.

> *"Just when the caterpillar thought the world was over it became a butterfly."*
> – English Proverb

I got to a new dark place or found myself suddenly at the bottom of the barrel, where I'd never expected or predicted I was on my road to that dead end road where I was forced to find an alternative route or else. I am here today to help you avoid getting to this roadblock suddenly in life as we do have "red flags" along the way that we may ignore or be "too busy" to even notice each day. I was forced to make changes- and till this day I am still recovering from the internal damage that I did to my body (hormones, gut infection and more) years later.

In this new existence, I roller-coasted from being a top long distance athlete who went from setting personal records and placing high in her age group and overall female in every race to gaining thirty pounds six months after Ironman Hawaii 2012 (which had nothing to do with what I was eating or my exercise sessions). I struggled with each pedal stroke up a gradual hill that used to be easy. I attempted to run under a ten-minute mile after racing at sub-eight-minute mile pace and I couldn't do it.

What happened to the happy, athletic, energetic endurance machine named Debbie Diesel?

I didn't recognize myself.

I was robbed… adrenal dysfunction stole my energy, self-esteem, confidence, endurance, power, toughness, and resiliency. My body simply would not respond anymore.

Three months after my last race in 2012 (North Face 50K trail run), I couldn't run without my heart rate going sky high and my legs feeling sluggish. I started waking up in the middle of the night (2:00 a.m. usually) with my mind wide alert. I had trouble remembering names and tasks I needed to complete each day. My bike rides became a challenge. My strong, powerful, cycling legs and endurance disappeared on the side of the road or maybe back in Kona.

Without any warning and pretty much what felt like overnight, I had these new rolls of fat—like a life preserver—was now on my waistline. New excess fat was now hanging over my waistband and on the back of my arms (which used to be my "best part" people said.) However, most noticeably for me was that my face got fuller and rounder. My "Debbie Arms" were gone and the fat tire around my waist was my new look.

I weighed myself in at the end June 2013 at a rental house in Coeur D'Alene during Ironman weekend to discover I had gained thirty unpleasant, shocking, freaking pounds. What the heck? Six months earlier, I was racing the North Face 50K in San Francisco and finishing a successful triathlon race season. Now, I was not able to fit in my clothes or walk around people without being embarrassed and ashamed of myself. Try running with a thirty-pound sandbag on your back. Thirty pounds is a lot. The only positive part of this share is I am tall (5' 10.5"), so the excess fat was spread around my tall long frame. Not as many people noticed—or so they said—as much as I did or felt. I was living in a different body. This was not the athletic fit happy me anymore.

Where did I lose myself along the way?

Where did the old me disappear to on the journey?

How did I go from kicking ass in a triathlon to melting down on the roadside during a simple bike ride?

Now, just because I did an excessive amount of training and racing over the years it wasn't the root to all of my health problems. Keep in mind that stress comes in different forms: good and bad. All stressors are funneled together in the body and processed the same way.

It could happen to anyone, not only an endurance athlete. Why? Because we all live each day as if we are participating in some type of long endurance race that doesn't have any rest stops or speed bumps along the way. We all sprint occasionally then recover to our own type of daily life interval training, but we go and go and go until we collapse into bed.

What is your daily battle?

We all handle chronic stress differently. You may be feeling like a winner and kicking booty each day closing deals, making a large bonus each quarter, nailing your financial or career goals, and attending every social event possible so you don't miss out on anything. Today you feel amazing, as I did only a few months prior to my internal breakdown. But, what is in your future? How long do you think you can tolerate a frenetic lifestyle and schedule? How many red flags, speed bumps, and signals to slow down that you have ignored from your central governor?

I was not as fortunate as you are today, as no one helped, stopped or warned me of what was coming in my future. I wasn't aware of my red flags that were being waved in my face for years prior to this event that was about to take place in 2013. I got caught up in the speed of life and I got my own type of "life speeding ticket" to force me to stop and change something immediately. You have one "get out of jail" card to use or else you are stuck on the hamster wheel of life. You only have one life… start to take ownership of yours.

I learned the hard way. Through sharing my story, you will see how if your adrenals are blown out and how the internal domino effect begins to all of your hormones and your main body systems.

Let me share my personal background so you can understand the experiences I had which brings me here today.

Burnout, Blow up, and Breakdown

2

"Sometimes you don't realize the weight of something you've been carrying until you feel the weight of its release."
– Power of Positivity

My story is told to help you see an example of the effects of how living each day as a race can catch up with you eventually. I found out the hard way. I want to help you avoid getting caught up in the speed of life, even if you are doing what you love. Sometimes it can be you're just trying to fit too much into one twenty-four hour period.

For me, I love training and racing for triathlons and being a competitive age group long distance triathlete as well as being a fitness studio owner, trainer, coach, and wife.

Back in my later twenties, my curiosity, research, education, and self-experimenting began to take over and I stopped relying on the mainstream media for my nutrition and health knowledge. Through self-learning and research, I discovered more about our body's metabolic efficiency, fat burning, sugar overload, and balancing hormones.

I have always been interested in nutrition and searching for the best food plan for myself. Why were some people able to eat anything and not gain weight even without exercising? Then, I would always be trying hard to "diet and exercise" to find the right solution for my body.

I wasn't really that overweight growing up, but I was not as petite or small as the other girls. Since my school years (mid-to-late 1980s), I was always on some new fad diet plan (like the soup diet) starting back as early as eight grade. Not only was I on some "magic diet" but I was going to the health club to working out for hours trying to lose weight. I went aerobics class after school or I went to work out on the Stairmaster and Nordic Track for an hour (while watching *The Cosby Show*, Thursday night TV) in the evening.

Obviously, I was into health and fitness at an early age, perhaps a little over the top for a few years in high school and into college. I suppose being a taller girl I always wanted to be "perfect" in order to fit in and have boys like me. I was too insecure and uptight about trying to change my looks. I knew back in high school I wanted to be teaching group exercise class as my 4:30 p.m. step aerobics instructor Nancy inspired me back in my high school days. I used to get to class early to be the class helper and ask her so many questions. A career in fitness was somehow going to be in my future but I had no idea how you make it a full-time job back in the eighties.

My high school senior year, I actually met weekly with a nutritionist at the club we were members of to help me eat healthier and lose a few pounds. This was my first, a probably last time; I kept a serious daily food log for at least six months. I was dedicated to eating exactly the right amount of food by measuring the amounts instructed by the nutritionist. During school, I wouldn't eat the food at lunch, only the pickles on the condiment bar. Then, I would do aerobics after school and for dinner, I would make a big salad. That was the tipping point in getting obsessed about what I ate and how I looked… and the beginning of damaging my metabolism. Yes, I lost weight by the old school way of eating less (only real food) and exercising more. Plus, I was finally getting more attention from the high school boys at the end of our senior year.

The fall of 1989 was a start of a new beginning as a freshman in college. Heading to college was the perfect opportunity to create my own identity. I was more confidence with my new lean body. The only problem was I didn't stop losing weight. First semester, I became so obsessed with only eating vegetables (amazing salad bar in the dorm cafeteria) while at Western Washington University in Bellingham, Washington. The Christmas break was an eye opener as one of my forever dear friends from high school called my parents to tell them she was worried about me. I was too skinny.

Constant dieting and eating low-calorie (processed "diet" foods) is another type of stress on our body. Not only are we feeding ourselves "non-foods," but we are always in emergency preservation mode. Yes, we need to teach our bodies how to burn fat instead of sugar, but there are more effective ways than eating the manufactured diet foods.

After that first year in college, my weight went the exact opposite way from being my lowest weight ever in my life (too low for sure) to the heaviest weight of my life (even with my adrenal dysfunction weight gain) a year later. I am sure these crazy years through the end of high school to the start of college impacted my metabolism, adrenals, and hormones. The stress of extreme body weight changes and low-calorie dieting followed by overeating only carbohydrates can drastically alter your hormones.

When I was in college, I continued being dedicated (or obsessed?) with working out each day. I was addicted to the endorphins or the mindset, apparently. Either way, I loved the feeling of exercise. After classes, I would head to the health club or aerobics studio or then head to the residence fitness center where I worked a few hours each day. From my college experience as the fitness coordinator on campus (the "Ridge"), I began to observe the personalities of the students that were into exercise, nutrition, and dieting.

We were all concerned about our body image and battled with self-esteem issues and exercise was a solution to improve it. I realized I wanted to help people with their health and fitness goals, challenges, obstacles, and struggles. I could relate to them. My fitness career as a trainer and coach began in my college years by working with the college students living in the dorms. My "birth" of a personal trainer and health coach started at an early age and much more fun that sticking with my original plan: business degree with a minor in French.

After graduation, I started working at a YMCA as a fitness and membership director to gain more experience. Then, I started working at the private health club where I grew up going to aerobics in the gym. Now, I was a fitness employee full-time at age twenty-five. My experience, observations, and the journey continued into the fueling, training, and performance for all levels athletes. Most people back then just want to lose weight, but now, my clients want to slow down the aging process as well as feel better and look better naked.

I started to think outside of the box about how I could lose weight and transform my body as well as my clients? While I was working as a personal trainer in my twenties (in the mid-1990s), *The Zone Diet* book came out. I started following it and attended seminars on nutrition. Through these classes, I understood my increased hunger levels after eating a high-carb "healthy" non-fat breakfast. In the early 2000s, *The Paleo Diet* book became a best seller. Now, I was beginning to comprehend the side effects of following a non-fat, high-carb food plan.

Even for an endurance athlete, it made no sense. The real confusion was for regular people wanting to lose ten to twenty pounds exercising more and eating less only provided short-term results.

When I was twenty-five-years-old, I discovered a new hobby and love: endurance events. Specifically, I was interested in long distance cyclings such as the Seattle to Portland Bike Ride and the Ride around Mr. Rainier in One Day (RAMROD) — both high-energy events. This was the start of my career as an endurance athlete. After I rode my first three-day bike ride, "The Tri-Island Bike Ride" for the American Lung Association, I knew I was going to be a cyclist. I rode my client's ex-husband's bike for the three-day event and with only training on a spin bike (I teach spin classes weekly), I was one of the first riders across the finish line for the day's ride. My legs and endurance were built for cycling and I loved riding outdoors in the country without busy streets, cars, traffic lights and stop signs ideally.

And, all of this led me to where I am today. To my business. My clients. My quest. My drive. My goals. But, also... my burn out.

Including my dedication and commitment to everything I do in life, I want to be successful in all areas, particularly in triathlons. On my way up to the top of the peak of the mountain, and before I fell quickly down the other side, I pushed myself as hard as I could. I ignored the stressors and red flags. It's no wonder I crashed like I did. Now, I can see how my constant racing was an additional interpreted stress by my brain/body even though I was having a blast and enjoying life as I knew how to best train and race.

Keep in mind that my triathlon coaches, Mark Allen and Luis Vargas, only gave me a training schedule for my "A" priority triathlons in the season (spring-fall) as well as the less important races used for training purposes (more what we classify as a "B" or "C" race). My off-season should have started in October and ended around February with cross-training and more focus on form, base training (low heart rate), and strength training while resting a bit more.

Typically, a triathlon season starts late spring or summer (depending on "A" race and location) and ends in September, unless you are doing the Ironman World Championship in October. When my Ironman season ended, usually with Ironman Hawaii, I started my "off-season" training, but it actually wasn't doing less endurance training as instructed by coaches. Mark Allen is very good at training athletes by heart rate (MAF training) and by time instead of miles, which is the ideal method not to over train and spend too much time in the "black hole" (long workout sessions above the aerobic max heart rate – or above anaerobic threshold area). I love training and racing, but I should have shut it down more in the fall and winter months.

For example… here is a glimpse of my race calendar for 2012-2013:

- January 2012: Carlsbad marathon
- May 2012: Vancouver half marathon
- July 2012: Lake Stevens 70.3 Triathlon; Hagg Lake Olympic Distance Triathlon
- August 2012: Ironman Canada (IMC) ("A" race to qualify); Personal Record (PR) on the bike 5:15 leg and

PR in Ironman. (Close to first place, but beat by a former Olympic swimmer who crushed me on the swim.)
- September 2012:
  - A week after Ironman Canada, there's no time to rest. Neal and I headed to Boulder, Colorado for Labor Day weekend to create workout videos with my coaches, Mark Allen and Luis Vargas, for their triathlon training website. While we were there, we had an amazing long uphill ride (my specialty) in the mountains from Boulder. Even though I just set a personal best time on the bike a week ago for IMC, my legs still felt amazingly fresh, strong , and fit on the long hill climb into the beautiful mountains; the ideal course for me. (So far so good. No red flags, yet.)
  - The next week, I had the 70.3 Ironman World Championships in Las Vegas with a swim in a dirty, man-made lake in 100-degree weather. My body was tired from Ironman Canada, but I was super happy and having fun. My focus turned to Kona. It was an incredibly hot day, but I was not being competitive and putting pressure on myself to place in my age group.
- October 2012: Hawaii Ironman World Championship – it was a windy day and I was a little slower than the previous year as I am sure fatigue had set in from my last two triathlons.
- November 2012: Marathon after doing an Ironman with a 2.4-mile swim, 112-mile bike, and a 26.2-mile run. Why didn't I just do a marathon (26.2 miles) by itself?

- December 2012: North Face 50k Trail Race – this was one of my favorite trail races in the Marin Headlands outside of San Francisco on the other side of the Golden Gate Bridge. My performance was strong, but not fast. This event was more about the journey and enjoying the amazing scenery and fresh clean air off the ocean and in the forest.
- January 2013: Carlsbad Marathon – I was seeing signs of fatigue setting in as my mile splits were not as fast as my past races, but I had to participate as it was an annual event I did with clients.
- February 2013: Chuckanut 50k trail race - my husband, Neal, had a great run, but he had to wait an hour for me to finish as I started to have big red flags with signs of fatigue and a high heart rate. This race was the start of me finally realizing something was wrong with me.
- March 2013: I tried to start my training for the "Honu 70.3" triathlon in June located in Kona, Hawaii. I had nothing in my legs or my overall tank. During my training for this race that never happened, I experienced the infamous breaking point meltdown, physical breakdown (and emotional) bike ride occurred. *Boom...* I am on the other side of the mountain with a quick slide from the peak down to the bottom, landing in a hole. My triathlon and race season was now over. End of my race season. I had to cancel my

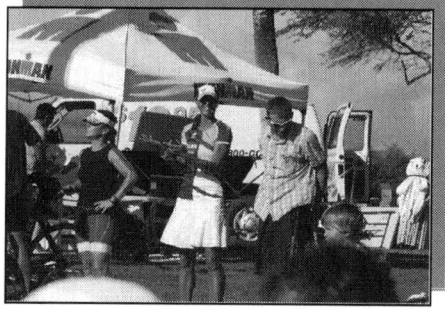

entry into both the "Honu 70.3" Triathlon and Ironman Canada races I had pre-registered for 2013.
- The transformation process begins. No more podium spots in 2013 or until... when?

Once my post-race depression disappeared, I always had the mentality that there was always a next time to set new time goals and break personal records (or so I thought I would have a next time.) Now, I struggle to run under 10:00-minute miles at my aerobic heart rate (MAF Formula 115-135 BMP). I once ran marathons under three hours and twenty minutes and half marathons under one hour and forty minutes. Once upon a time, I was able to average a 7:30-mile pace for a marathon (26.1 miles), but now that is a distant memory.

As people say "back in the day," I managed to run 26.2 miles at the end of an Ironman (after swimming 2.4 miles and biking 112 miles) faster than I could run a 5K today. Slightly depressing, yes. The days of running a 3:12 marathon in Boston seem like a lifetime away.

Do I think my races in 2012 were my "glory days" as a triathlete? Now, I am an "aging athlete" and slower because of the aging process? I disagree. What happened, you wonder? Doing too much became toxic. It doesn't matter that I was doing too many races- it was the additional time I added to my already busy schedule as a business owner, trainer, coach, and wife. I literally added the hours of another part-time job on top of a full-time job.

You may not be doing an Ironman and/or a marathon, but you could be running a company or your own household plus juggling school activities, board meetings, and volunteer jobs on top of a full-time job. More is not always better.

Perhaps you can predict what was going to happen or not

as we are often oblivious to doing too much and determining how much too much for the body. You can only be at your peak performance and ask your body of so much for only so long before it breaks down. Too much of anything can be toxic and interpreted in the body (HPA Axis) as stress. Too much training, racing, and what is termed chronic cardio is toxic to the body.

When you are on an endurance junkie "high," you don't realize that "more is less" and often toxic to your body. I was happy and enjoying life, so why not do what I loved to do in life which was training and racing for a triathlon?

I planned to do my usual recovery period in November and December to help recover from 2012 race season and then start to rebuild for the next triathlon race season in 2013. After finishing the 2012 season with personal best times (PRs) and placing top in my age group as well as overall in each race, I was I was confident and determined to reach my new overall time goal for Ironman Canada 2013 with a 10:15 finishing time. If you believe in your ability and visualize a goal, you can achieve it. Right? I had received a fridge magnet from Ironman Hawaii with the numbers you can create your new goal. To this day, the time goal magnet is still on the fridge with the time of 10:15 for Ironman 2013.

The year of 2013 was underway as planned, but I gradually began to feel a little off. I wasn't recovering from my workouts. I will admit my "off season" that year did not include slowing down and resting. I felt I was fit and in peak condition so why not do a marathon since running 26.2-miles was a piece of cake after doing two full Ironmans.

My husband and I did our annual 50K trail event/race we love in the Marin Headlands outside of San Francisco. The North Face 50K includes lots of walking for me so I figured my heart rate would be low enough and it was a long hike, so why not do a 50k if I have the endurance and strength?

Of course, I had to do the Carlsbad Marathon in January as I always trained a group of clients for the Carlsbad half or full marathon (beautiful course along the coast). Why not? I was invincible.

Neal and I did one more "off season" training event which was a 50K trail run in Bellingham, Washington (Chuckanut 50K) in February. For some unknown reason, my heart rate was running higher at the same pace so I had to slow down and walk. The trail run event including a lot more walking for me to keep my heart rate in my aerobic range, but I was so much slower than normal that Neal was sitting in the car waiting for me for an hour wondering why I was taking so long. Red flag.

I tried to take it "easy," but obviously I don't rest well. I prefer what I call "active recovery" instead of simply taking a week off without any exercise. Maybe I needed more actual rest. In March, I was in Spokane, Washington for Ben Greenfield's Superhuman Conference where we had speakers talk on Heart Rate Variability and Adrenal dysfunction. As one of the "Superhuman Coaches," my friend, Brock, and I led one of the morning group runs. I was not feeling strong and my heart rate was high. Something was going on. Maybe I was overtraining, but I usually bounced back after races and training sessions.

However, a major awakening occurred in April on a training bike ride...

I will never forget this day.

I was on a typical longer bike ride with my husband, Neal, and one of our training partner friends, Joel. I can visualize the entire segment of the bike ride where the breakdown occurred. This wasn't a bike mechanical issue; this was a Debbie breakdown—physically and emotionally. This was hitting the rock bottom. I knew for sure that something bad was going on.

On a Saturday in April 2013, we were riding from our house to Black Diamond, Washington for a typically easy fifty miles through rolling hills. Suddenly, I couldn't keep pedaling or spinning my legs. They simply wouldn't work and I had no energy to do even one pedal stroke. My muscles were not firing and they were fighting back. My body said, "Enough! I'm done!"

So, I had to pull over. I yelled ahead to Neal and Joel that I had to stop for a moment and then the tears started pouring out. I was scared and confused.

What was wrong with my leg strength and my energy? I couldn't keep up with my husband and Joel when I was always a strong cyclist. I had a meltdown on the side of the road, then tried to ride ahead to let them know I had to turn around and head back home. I didn't have a flat tire; *I* was flat physically.

The boys rode ahead and I took the easy way home. I was afraid I was not able to get all the way there even when taking the flat Cedar River trail. How could I suddenly be on the top of my game and then have nothing; no muscle strength or endurance to pedal any further? I wanted to scream, yell, cry, and throw my bike into the bushes. First, I had to get home.

I'd just finished the best racing year of my life (2012) and suddenly 2013 was gearing up to be the worst of my career. I had to start wondering if the 2012 triathlon season was the end of my career. Was Kona my last Ironman triathlon and my last time qualifying for Worlds?

I wonder if this breakdown, blow up, and burn out was some type of payback from the universe for never stopping to pause and reset and for also never being grateful for my accomplishments in life and sports. I was never satisfied with my race results even when I was on the podium as a top finisher plus it was rare that I shared my race success with my clients and friends. I was a "closet" racer; no bragging or sharing my podium finishes. I was always embarrassed to wear an Ironman finisher shirt or merchandise, nevertheless get a popular tattoo (IM) that many triathletes got after their first IM finish. I was very humble about my race history and "resume," but that is how I was and still would be today. Maybe I should be more celebratory of my success, especially now.

My "wellness bank account" was robbed. I had too many withdrawals and not enough deposits in my account. I loved training and racing for Ironman triathlons, but at what cost? Everyone is different how many types of life stressors they can tolerate. I went overboard in the way I lived my daily life with running a business, training my clients, coaching athletes, financial stress, then adding too much intermittent fasting and too many hours training: triathlon training plus yoga, strength training, and hours teaching group training, spin class, and run group.

I tried to do more of everything in a twenty-four hour day and take care of everyone which resulted in less quality sleeping. I thought I was having fun, being happy, and enjoying my life, but I was trying to do too much.

One day, I felt incredibly fit, unbeatable, and tough and almost overnight and very shockingly unexpectedly, I was extremely fatigued, exhausted, and broken down from the inside out. I could not understand what happened to me in March 2013 right after I was setting my personal best triathlon times, running a busy fitness studio, and feeling amazing on a daily basis. I thought my life was on the right track and I was going to be successful since I was organized, productive, and always busy.

My body was telling me something else. A few hints filled with negative feedback. I was forced to wonder if this "meltdown" or "burnout" I was experiencing was a result of my excessive training or my lifestyle.

When I started college, I had no idea exercise science was actually a degree so, of course, I started my secondary education going the business route as everyone else I knew was taking business courses. I quickly figure out that wasn't my thing. So, I looked into a nutrition degree, but that was too much chemistry. I went into the recreation program thinking I wanted to do tourism and hotel management since I liked people and loved to travel. Nope, that wasn't enough. I finally discovered exercise science courses then supplemented them with health education and immediately found my calling. The exercise science courses interested me. Unexpectedly, I was the fitness coordinator for the college dorms and running fitness orientations, fitness challenges, as well as running the aerobics classes. That was the start of my fitness career back in 1991 at Western Washington University in Bellingham, Washington.

When I exercise, especially outside on my bike or when running, I feel refreshed, happy, and relaxed. Perhaps it is just getting out in the outdoors, breathing the fresh air, seeing the bright blue sky, and the feeling warmth of the sunshine. How can that be bad for your health? Now, I understand a lot more. It has taken me over three years to figure out my problems or triggers to the health problems I continue to heal from. The accumulation of everything I was doing, every day, all day, was taking a toll of on my health as my brain interpreted what I thought was healthy for me as a type of stress. I was in "emergency mode" constantly. My cruise control button was on from the time I woke up until I went back to bed. I thought I needed to rest more, to recover longer, and to cut down on my triathlon and running races as well as events.

I now understand more about the HPA Axis—the communication system from the brain to the pituitary gland to the adrenal glands was becoming exhausting, like a circuit breaker blowing up and becoming dysfunctional (the inability to function; "failing to perform an expected function" or, simply put, "out of order" until repaired.)

How could I be breaking down my body when I was training in my low heart rate training range (Max Aerobic Function training = MAF -more later) and eating a low-carb real food plan where I thought I was avoiding the risk of high heart rating training as Dr. Maffetone writes about (a must read article for endurance athletes): But, I wasn't really doing any high heart rate intensity training or intervals- or eating processed foods. I was doing a high volume of training... plus leading a busy life every day with a full schedule.

> *"Excess high training intensity or training volume and/or excess consumption of processed/refined dietary carbohydrates can contribute to reduced health in athletes and even impair performance."*
> *- Unknown*

Read more at: http://tinyurl.com/spingeropen

The term MAF means maximum aerobic function. MAF training is ideal for anyone striving to improve optimal performance. Athletes of all levels, as well as for those who want to reduce body fat and improve athletic function. The MAF type of training fit perfectly into The WHOLESTIC Method - one of the eight elements is the type of exercise to burn fat, optimize health (reduce stress), and improve performance.

My workouts to this day are my when I actually relax and get into a "Zen" mindset. My creative brain works and I solve the world's problems (or min, as least). I didn't want to believe my weekly dedicated training program could be the culprit of my exhaustion and lack of recovery from workouts, but then other symptoms occurred. I couldn't figure out what the rhyme or reason was to my sudden onset of multiple random unusual health problems I was now experiencing day after day.

Today, I can finally look at the big picture of my exhaustion and internal breakdown of my body's systems and how they are related to the way I lived my WHOLE entire life, not only my exercise, but my way of operating day to day tasks. I realized I was always intense and focused with everything I did. However, being intense also means being tense.

My creative brain waves were at work while I exercise. This is actually the "alpha brain waves" which I'll discuss more in The WHOLESTIC Method Manual in the chapter on sleep.

> *"Alpha waves (8 to 12 Hz) are present when your brain is in an idling default-state typically created when you're daydreaming or consciously practicing mindfulness or meditation. Alpha waves can also be created by doing **aerobic exercise.**"*

Source: http://tinyurl.com/alphabrainwaves

I woke up at 3:45 a.m. to arrive at my studio (Fitness Forward Studio) to check emails before clients arrived around 5:15 a.m. That was only the start and my day and it didn't end until around 7:00 p.m. most days. How about being addicted to being busy?

Perhaps my overscheduled days and busy lifestyle were a major factor in my (adrenal) hormonal and body systems break down or fall out. The circuit breaker finally blew up.

Could that be it?

I mean, who else was to blame but me?

I continue to recover from my health problems that followed this breakdown. I was forced to make some changes. It wasn't until I sat down to write my story that I realized my brain doesn't turn off. I am always "working" on something. To be still and simply relax to empty the mind as if in a meditative state is challenging to me which is why my magic place I go to unplug, let go, and relax in my mind is Kona, Hawaii.

We often need to embrace change and see a transformation into someone new is a wonderful thing; not depressing or a negative experience.

To completely understand my fall, burn out, blow out, and ultimate disappointment, let me take you through the exhilarating experience of an Ironman competition, what happens, how you feel, what you experience, and that adrenaline high when you cross the finish line…

The Thrill of Victory 3

*"So often we become so focused on the finish line
that we fail to enjoy the journey."*
– Dieter F. Uchtdorf

In October 2012, I was at the start line of the Ironman World Championships in Kona, Hawaii. This was my fifth time qualifying for the World Championships.

The big show of the Ironman race series.

Each year, the Ironman comes to a close with the Ironman World Championship Triathlon in Kona, Hawaii. Ironman Hawaii is the triathlon most all competitive Ironman triathletes strive to qualify for each year (if you qualify for Ironman Hawaii after October, then you are guaranteed a slot in the following year's World Championship race).

You are known as a bad ass if you qualify for the Hawaii Ironman World Championships. I didn't think that about myself until after the fact. You must qualify for the World Championship by placing in the top three in your age group (which is a difficult feat to achieve and a major accomplishment in the Ironman world).

My Ironman triathlon career started in 2001, at age twenty-nine and I quickly fell in love with the training and the race experience. In 2012, I was having the best race season of my triathlon career and I was placing top in my age group and overall in Olympic distance triathlons, half Ironmans and with the full Ironman distance triathlon. The distance of an Ironman triathlon is a daunting 2.4-mile swim, 112-mile bike, and a 26.2-mile run, but when you cross the finish line and hear the phrase,

"You are an IRONMAN" on the overhead speakers, you don't think about how many miles you did any more to get to the finish line. At Ironman Hawaii 2012, the World Championship, I had no idea what was going to happen around six months later and I had no idea this could have been my last Ironman triathlon.

Leading up to Kona, the World Championships for Ironman, I was in the best fitness and racing shape of my life. In each triathlon I participated in 2012, the time I ran a race or triathlon; I was setting personal best times and placing in my age group. My type of training had paid off after years of focusing on training by heart rate (MAF) and changing my eating habits to a lower carb/higher fat plan. The training plan helped me to become a metabolically efficient athlete or a fat-burning machine. The end result was my improved ability to bike and run faster while staying in my aerobic heart rate ranges where I was still burning lots of fat for fuel instead of sugar.

As I look back to my www.athlinks.com race records, I was pulling off a 7:17 pace per mile in a half-marathon, placing first in my age group in Olympic distance triathlons, which was way faster than the pace I currently run today. Every race I was strong, faster, and focused, including half Ironmans, half-marathons, and—my proudest moment—finishing Ironman distance in Penticton, British Columbia, Canada with my fastest time since my Ironman career started in 2001.

After crossing the finish line in Ironman Canada at 10:22:55 with a personal best bike split of 5:17:27, I was on cloud nine and happy while feeling calm and relaxed when racing strong at a fast pace. From my exercise and eating style, I had created what is called a "metabolically efficiency" system. I could burn high amounts of fat at higher heart rates and long distance endurance events were comfortable for me. My body was so metabolically efficient that I could ride so at faster speeds while keeping my heart rate aerobic (with oxygen-burning fat), yet still feel relatively comfortable and still be able to cheer on my fellow participants racing around me (with a big smile on my face in my happy place).

From years of aerobic (endurance-burn fat-use oxygen; I can go forever pace) zone training, I had built up my "MAF" aerobic max training ranges (180-age) (see MAF Formula in The WHOLESTIC Method manual) and turned my fat burning engine on overdrive. I could train at or around 150 heart rates or beats per minute (BPM) and still burning mostly fat for fuel instead of sugar.

From my years of building up my aerobic engine (building my foundation) with my endurance training (I started distance events as cycling back in 1996), I became very metabolically efficient, which meant I could burn fat at higher heart rates and avoid the typical "bonking"—where you feel you are hitting the wall due to racing anaerobically (lack of oxygen) which you can only maintain for so long before being exhausted. With my proper training schedule from Mark Allen, I continued to increase my speed or pace on my bike and running while maintaining the same aerobic heart rates (breathing comfortably) around 130-150 heart rates or BMP. By not going into anaerobic heart rate ranges—or without oxygen—I was able to utilize fat as my main fuel source for long periods of time and not get exhausted… when training and racing. More about metabolic efficiency later.

Brooks Running Company uses the slogan "Run Happy." I like to use the phrase "Race Happy" as it always will leave you with a positive race day experience. I always prefer competing with a smile on my face. Smiling, laughing, and keeping positive resulted in racing happy (one of The WHOLESTIC Method elements) I was sharing, or rather paying forward, my energy and enthusiasm to the other athletes in the race to help inspire and motivate. By cheering my fellow Ironman Canada participants by their first name (names on the race numbers on their back) while we were on the bike leg then the run leg allowed me to keep on my endorphin high while helping others have fun and enjoy the experience – the journey.

Happiness is contagious as we discuss in my manual, The WHOLESTIC Method. One of my eight secrets to burning fat, optimizing health, and improving performance is HAPPINESS. I talk about the "10-5 Rule" in my manual which I apply to my bike and run workouts, as well as raceS… my abundance of joy and thrill of excitement of racing was contagious to my fellow triathletes friends for over ten hours.

I realize most people would wonder how can swim 2.4-miles, biking 112-miles and then running 26.2-miles be fun? When I train and race, I get in the Zen mindset and feel a peace… my happy place. When you are relaxed, at ease, and confident in your abilities, (and potential) I told myself, "No one can beat me. I am strong, I am fast, and I am powerful." At least, I was the only one who had to believe in my abilities. A positive mindset and confidence in your abilities in life—any type of "race" you may experience—is essential in order to enjoy the journey we are experiencing at this present moment. Instead, many people begin their race or event with negativity, stress, and anxiety that does more harm than good in most cases.

Getting back to Ironman Canada, at the end of the race, I completed my celebratory finish line push-ups, (one for each completed Ironman) and then my typical post-race nausea (always predictable once my body stopped moving). My fellow new triathlon friends crossed the finish line, and then (I was cheering them on during the bike leg of the race) stopped by to thank me for keeping them motivating and continuing to race strong. I paid my happiness forward to others around me and it was quite rewarding.

Toward the end of the 112-mile bike ride at the top of Yellow Lake, one of the volunteers yelled out that I was one of the top ten females overall. *Overall?* Wow! Now *that* got me more fired up to finish strong. I cruised to the bike finish in Penticton and raced through the transition area to start the last part of the race with full-out gusto and vigor. The remainder was a 26.2-mile run out and back along the beautiful Okanagan lakes.

My husband/best friend/training partner, Neal, was on the course right at the beginning of the run course. He told me my bike split was a 5:17 and there was only one person in front of me to catch. She was an Olympic athlete. *What?* I'd felt amazingly strong and fast on the bike while never pushing myself out of my comfort level and staying within my aerobic training ranges (burn fat for fuel so you last longer = metabolic efficiency.) I was in shock that I pulled off a 5:17 bike split, so I was fired up to run strong and relaxed to hope to catch the "Olympian" (not saying her name yet) on the run. My strength is my bike ride, so my goal is to always get a head start on the run and avoid the strong entrants running me down. This time, it was my turn to run the first place girl down in front of me.

The IM Canada race course was in Penticton, B.C. in the beautiful Okanogan. Sadly, this was the last year of this race that had been held here for thirty years, so I wanted to experience my best race ever as this course was made for me. The run was out 13.1-miles then a turn-around to head to the finish line. The first half of the race, a half-marathon (13.1-miles), I felt comfortable and then my mindset was to start another "half marathon" and race it after "Mile 8" or near the start of town. Thankfully, Neal was out on the course keeping me focused and going, even though I yelled at him to stop talking to me as I ran in my "zone." Plus, the other race participants were running out the other direction on the first half of the course, so I had other cheerleaders to inspire and motivate me to finish strong.

Now, I didn't know who this Olympian was ahead of me. Of course, I wanted to catch her as I wanted to be the first place finisher. My amazingly supportive husband, Neal, was out on the run course (via his bike) to give me updates on how far ahead "she" was and how much I was gaining on her. My goal is to always run relaxed and happy. If I push myself too hard too early, then I will blow up. So, I am faithful to my heart rate ranges I know I can maintain without going anaerobic (not enough oxygen and you burn sugar) and wear out too early. Instead, I am very good at pacing myself (ironic) in a race and building up my pace to the end. This is one of the secrets to my success as an endurance athlete as I am taller (5' 10.5") and not small. I can ride strong and hold my own on the run.

Neal finally told me during the second half of the run the girl in my age group who was in first place and I was trying to catch all day was the ex-Olympic swimmer, Susan Williams.

Still, in my head, I thought, "This race is mine." What does an Olympic swimmer have on me, someone racing in her fourteenth Ironman? Even though I had a swim start that threw me off my time goals (off by five minutes of my average IM swim splits), I ran as fast as I could to the finish line in Penticton. It is one of those annoying finish lines where you have to run past the finish area to do another mile then turn down to the finish chute. I finished with a smile on my face, but I was second place.

There were my amazing results with a personal record (PR) for overall time and bike split, but all I noticed was one thing. My swim split. If I'd swam my best average 1:05 to 1:08 time for Penticton swim split, I could have been first place age group (AG) winner.

> Potts, Deborah BELLEVUE WA USA
> **134** OVERALL out of 2423 finishers
> Finishing time: 10:22:58
> W40-44 Age group: 2/168
> Swim Split: 30 AG/874 overall/1:13:23 time split/1:56 pace per 100m. Transition One: 3:11
> Bike Splits: 1st Age group/ 119 overall/5:17:27 time/21.2 average speed; Transition 2: 2:14
> Run: 4th best in AG/ 158 overall/ 3:46:46 time/8:40 average pace

As a typical type-A personality athlete, I always feel I could have done better even though I just completed my best overall Ironman (IM) finishing time and bike split. As predicted, my endorphin high post-race excitement of finishing my best overall IM time was immediately overpowered by my disappointment in my swim results. My mood transitioned into my predictable post-race depression; never satisfied or appreciative of my success and instead, dwelling on the negative or rather "my areas of opportunity" (mentally positive phrase to say what you are weak at or need improvement). Rather than making the situation into something positive, I was quick to turn it around into a negative experience. However, it was only one hour plus of the over ten hour race day.

Why are we so hard on ourselves even when we are performing at our very best?

Every week for years, I've worked on my swim stroke during masters swim workout or lessons (I need more private lessons.) But lesson learned (the hard way) don't ask for help before a race. I made a major mistake getting swim technique advice from a friend a few days before my major "A" race (IM Canada). Big mistake. Over-focusing on your swim stroke will make you slower rather than faster, at least, that is my personal opinion (and experience).

Another source of stress was trying too hard to be perfect or get faster in a sport when you probably just need to relax, quiet your mind, and settle down. Slow and smooth. All I could think about now was if I swam my usual 1:05 to 1:08 Ironman 2.4 mile swim split, then I would/could/should have placed first in my age group instead of second which was a major bummer and emotional setback. My personal triathlon race goals are to always to beat my previous time splits (swim, bike, and run) as well as my overall (OA) finisher time than my previous races.

I had severe post-race depression and extremely disappointed in my race performance. Even though I had an absolutely amazing personal best Ironman Canada bike split (5:17) and run (3:46) times, I was still unhappy and dissatisfied with my overall race performance- just because of my slower swim. How sad is that? If I only knew now what I knew then, I would be on cloud nine. However, my competitive mindset was, "I can do better." Next time.

I reminisce now and I am disappointed at myself for not celebrating the fact that I was second in my age group (as well as runner-up to a former Olympic athlete swimmer). Oh, how I wish I would have been more grateful for my successes instead of looking at the negatives. I never reviewed my results or bragged about them- until now! Plus I am not sure if I will be able to race Ironman again -especially since that Ironman Canada is no longer in Penticton.

> Fastest Bike - Age Group Women
> Place/Bike/Number/Name City Pro Cnt
> 1 5:16:48 2180 Lee, Kendra DENVER CO
> **2 5:17:27 2476 Potts, Deborah BELLEVUE WA**
> 3 5:17:35 2416 Scaroni, Pia SAN FRANCI CA

This should not be depressing, but it is. I forgot my finishing time as I never appreciated what I'd accomplished until now as I write about my journey.

> Women 40 - 44 Awards
> Place Time Number Last Name First Name Age City Pro Cnt
> Swim Tr1 Bike Tr2 Run
> 1 10:18:26 2560 Williams, Susan 43 LITTLETON CO USA 53:15/ 2:45/ 5:29:15/ 2:53/ 3:50:19
> **2 10:22:58 2476 Potts, Deborah 41 BELLEVUE WA USA 1:13:23/ 3:11/ 5:17:27/ 2:14/ 3:46:46**

My 2.4-mile IM swim split in Penticton Ironman Canada in 2012 was actually my worst performance (swim time) of my triathlon racing career. My only other horrible swim, besides the IM Hawaii ocean swim, was the time I almost drowned in Ironman Coeur D'Alene because of hyperventilating due to the cold water. (Listen to my podcast on Swimming for Triathlons for listed in the resource section at the end of the book.) Susan Williams did one of the best swims of the day with an amazing 53:15 split compared to my lollygagging, over rotating, over trying to swim a new stroke with super slow (for me) 1:13 split. That is all I focused on... until now. It is possible to over focus on one element of an experience and not being so hard on ourselves.

I over-analyze and do the "could have/should have" stories in my head. Ideally, I would have caught her on the bike if I had gotten out of the water ten minutes faster than I did (don't try to over-rotate when swimming or be too much in a Zen state.) I was too focused on my freestyle swim stroke technique and body positioning and staying relaxed which only resulted in going slower. The slower swimmers were passing me as I looked around. Slower meant slower. I needed to find that happy balance in between picking up my pace without rushing my swim stroke. That was all I thought about days after that Ironman triathlon. Boo hoo... get out the violin. Pity party for one. I was feeling sorry for myself instead of celebrating my accomplishments in the big picture. We are always our worst enemy when we should be our own biggest cheerleader.

Now, I only share my best race results for you to create the dramatic effect of what was about to happen in my near future as the chapter is called "from bad ass to fat ass" (okay only in my eyes and personal opinion). The lesson learned from my 2012 race (and life) experiences was to be more grateful, appreciative, and thankful. I wish I would have been more appreciative for the athletic abilities, metabolic efficiency and aerobic engine that I had built up over the years (learn more about metabolic efficiency in my exercise chapter in The WHOLESTIC Method manual).

We take what we have for granted and we don't appreciate something (or someone) until we lose it. I wish we would all live each day without any regrets as we never know what tomorrow will bring... the "present" is a gift, but why don't we always realize that and be grateful? Sometimes, we don't realize how good life is until the parts come tumbling down (or comes unraveled) as my health overnight (but in reality months).

After my amazing race experience and achievement of setting a new personal best overall finishing time (besides my super slow swim.) at Ironman Canada in Penticton, B.C. 2012, I continued to feel strong, powerful and in peak condition during my training sessions. At another half Ironman (70.3 triathlon) in Lake Stevens, WA, in June 2012, I qualified for the Ironman 70.3 World Championships again to be held in Vegas in September 2012. However, doing yet another long distance triathlon race after I just completed the Ironman Canada triathlon two weeks prior to World 70.3 in Vegas was a bit much, but I had to do the race as it was so close to home. I still had my "A" race (biggest priority) Ironman Hawaii World Championships in a few weeks after Vegas 70.3 Worlds.

Why not do another major triathlon championship race and go on one more trip? I was feeling fit, strong, and invincible. My mindset was that I would treat 70.3 World Championship in Las Vegas as a "training" day and use it as a practice session (race simulator) for my main "A" priority triathlon race in Kona, Hawaii- the Ironman World Championship that next October. That was a lot of racing within 6-8 weeks.

After an extremely hot 105-degree Ironman 70.3 distance triathlon "training" day in Las Vegas, I could tell my body needed a break; recovery time to heal and rebuild. If I was going to be rested and ready for Ironman World Championship, I had to force myself to back off my training schedule for a few weeks- recover and rest more.

Rest? What is rest?

I was motivated and focused on recovering in time to be ready again to race the most challenging Ironman Triathlon course of them all -and the toughest competitive field of top age group and professional athletes from around the world.

The Ironman World Championship is the dream for most triathletes, including me, to experience and earn a qualification spot. I started racing Ironman triathlons in 2001 and after I started being coached by the Ironman legend, Mark Allen, and joining the Mark Allen Elite Team in 2003, I started qualifying for Ironman Hawaii World Championship race each year. Keep in mind; you have to qualify in another Ironman triathlon that same year by placing first to third in your age group (depending on how many slots are available in the specific IM race). Since I qualified in 2012 at Ironman Canada at the end of August (not ideal race to qualify in as you don't have enough recovery time in between races), I had only six weeks to prepare (or recover) for another Ironman, but this one was the World Championship you see on television (or rather the dramatic, edited down, tinkly piano music version NBC provides for viewers to make them cry.).

So, what is the IRONMAN and how did it start?

"The inaugural Hawaiian IRONMAN Triathlon was conceptualized in 1977 as a way to challenge athletes who had seen success at endurance swim, running and biathlon events. Honolulu-based Navy couple, Judy and John Collins, proposed combining the three toughest endurance races in Hawai'i—the 2.4-mile Waikiki Rough water Swim, 112 miles of the Around-O'ahu Bike Race and the 26.2-mile Honolulu Marathon—into one event. On February 18, 1978, fifteen people came to Waikiki to take on the IRONMAN challenge. Prior to racing, each received three sheets of paper with a few rules and a course description. The last page read: "Swim 2.4-miles. Bike 112-miles. Run 26.2-miles. Brag for the rest of your life. In 1981, the race moved from the tranquil shores of Waikiki to the barren

lava fields of Kona on the Big Island of Hawai'i. Along the Kona Coast, black lava rock dominates the panorama, and athletes battle the "ho'omumuku" crosswinds of forty-five miles per hour, ninety-five-degree temperatures, and a scorching sun. The IRONMAN World Championship centers on the dedication and courage exhibited by participants who demonstrate the IRONMAN mantra that ANYTHING IS POSSIBLE.® Each year athletes will embark on a 140.6-mile journey that presents the ultimate test of body, mind, and spirit to earn the title of IRONMAN.

Source: http://tinyurl.com/IronmanCompetitions

Kona, Hawaii is where Ironman World Championship ("Worlds" for short) is held every October. The small town of Kona is taken over by obnoxious (my opinion.) top age group triathletes from around the world. I love the energy and vibe, especially people watching, *but* it can also be extremely intimidating as these are the best triathletes who earned a spot in the top Ironman race.

You can watch all sorts of triathletes walk around town in their speedos, especially after the morning warm-up swims at the pier at "Dig-I beach." Then, all day you will see triathletes exercising the few days up to the race day (the second Saturday of October) on the run course along Ali'i Drive and biking too much on the Queen K highway. Triathletes are typically all type-A personalities; those who always do too much. We are not good a sitting around and being still, but Mark Allen taught me a lot about calming the mind and resting. Actually, Kona, Hawaii is one of the only places I really unwind, unplug, and let go. I can work out in the morning, then sit on the beach or by the pool as long as I can watch the wave's crash into the shoreline. Kona is my magic place where I can feel the healing of the island.

If you have ever been to Kona, you know the wind is always a major factor when training and especially on race day. Those trade winds are constantly throwing out surprises and catching triathletes off guard when cycling along the Ironman Hawaii bike course through the lava fields on the Queen K and the beautiful road to Hawi. One must be prepared for various weather conditions like the heat, headwinds, tailwind, and severe side winds.

How does this relate to life, though?

Well, Mother Nature is always unpredictable in our daily existence.

In order to survive and conquer the Ironman Hawaii bike course, as well as in our own daily life, we need to have relative flexibility and not be so rigid. Relative flexibility is the ability to change and cope with variable circumstances or, more specifically, how our body tends to seek a path of least resistance whenever moving.

We need to be capable of adjusting our workout or our work schedule to meet the demands of Mother Nature and what she is throwing at us on a daily basis. In other words, in order to avoid exhausting our stress response system- including our adrenal glands from all forms of accumulative and chronic stress, we need to be able to have resilience and be capable of withstanding any type of stress that comes our way without damage to our overall health.

Sometimes, we need to compromise and work with what we have right now. The Kona trade winds are an example of one of those tests we face as an Ironman triathlete.

For Ironman World Championship race day, I needed to put on the best performance of my life as one would be surrounded by the top age groupers from around the world. I wanted to be one of the top ten people in the 40-44 age groups in the world. I felt confident this was my year to be top ten since I was coming off an amazing race season and setting my best times at each event.

The week leading up to race day is always exciting and busy at the same time with the buzz in town, race expo, parade, and opening ceremonies dinner. Plus, we always had our "Mark Allen Elite" team breakfast where our head coach, Mark Allen, would give us his speech to help us stay calm, focused, and mentally strong for the task ahead of us as the Island is predictable.

The weather—the heat and the wind—is always a factor and the main element to break an athlete on race day. The swells in the ocean for the swim can be powerful, the crosswinds and side winds on the bike are always changing, and then the heat on the bike and during the run steaming off the pavement can be unbearable.

The bike along the Queen K highway is long, but busy with other cyclists all on the same mission: to get to the turnaround in Hawi, then head toward the transition area before the winds (and heat) pickup later in the day. The winds in Kona are always changing and unpredictable, just as we will discuss later. That is another reason I love Kona; you never know what Mother Nature will offer you at that moment or what the island gods will present you.

The run turnaround is called the "Energy Lab." This is the point of the race where people can overheat, as well as struggle physically and mentally. The heat can melt you down from the inside out, but I often find the "Energy Lab" motivating as you do the out-and-back portion of the run, then head back on the Queen K to the most amazing finishing lines in the world. The cruise down "Pay-n-Save" hill is exciting as you reach the last mile of the Ironman World Championship, then the goosebumps and smiles come out after a long hot challenging day at the office.

I absolutely *love* the last run onto to Ali'i Drive toward the finish chute under my favorite tree (you know it if you have been there) to run fast as you can to the IM Finish line. The body is amazing no matter how exhausted you are physically and emotionally; it will work when you see the finish line in Kona.

That finish line is why we race another Ironman to qualify for the World Championship in Kona, Hawaii. Crossing the finish line in Kona is an unbelievable and magical experience.

Race day in Kona for the World Championship is always unpredictable. The weather is always changing, even on race day. When you are racing Ironman Hawaii on the bike segment, you are not in control of the conditions (wind and heat) and almost everyone will have a different experience. For example, the weather for the professionals (who begin before the age groupers) will have different wind conditions in the swim, then on the run as the wind seems to always shift directions every few minutes... or hour.

Every year, the Ironman Hawaii the race course is the same, but the wind is always different. One year could be large swells in the swim then a headwind on the bike then side winds, then more headwinds. Somehow, I rarely felt tail winds which give you some "free" speed. You can go faster on the bike with less effort but those headwinds or side winds are brutal- and similar to climbing hills. My point is that the ever-shifting weather conditions on the Big Island of Hawaii are always challenging your mindset, patience, and confidence – the unpredictability with Mother Nature on this magical island is similar to our daily life.

We can't stress about what we can't have control over and we need to learn how to be more resilient to unpredictable situations or experiences in order to survive life (at least if we stay healthy in life). The Ironman Hawaii race experience not only challenges your physical talent and strengths, but also your mental strength… which is why I find Kona my healing place as I always leave the island feeling stronger on the inside and out and ready to deal with my hectic daily life.

To race Ironman Hawaii, you must be able to also quiet the mind and learn how to let go negative talk in your head (as in any race or life event.). We all need to learn how to quiet the negative self-talk and child ego to bring out the positive attitude and improve self-esteem required for surviving daily life responsibilities, obligations and expectations (of society).

After waiting patiently on the Kona Pier transition area, we line up in the ocean at the deep water swim start. Before the swim warm up and start line (always a challenge feeling like a human bobble head in the ocean swells), we go through another process you can call "pre-race" set up. Usually, I arrive at the start line two hours before the race (7:00 a.m. for IM) to allow enough time to set up my transition area as well as get body marking. The body marking process at IM Worlds is always entertaining to me. Before the new race number "tattoos" they use at most races now, our race numbers would be stamped with ink on our arms and our age was on our calf (sadly they stopped stamping your age. I loved to see who was in my age group when racing). Once we were stamped, we would then follow the cattle call to the swimming pier where we would have our bike set up at a specific spot based on your race number. The day before the race, we set up our bike and did a sort of "walk through" of the transition area. This is ideal if you want to have smooth transitions from the swim to the bike to the run.

The day before the race, as well as the morning of, all triathletes (only ones allowed in transition area) need—or rather should—to rehearse where we get out of the ocean after the swim to grab your "T1" bike bag then changing tent back to our bike. This is called transition one or for short "T1." After T1, we need to practice heading out to the bike start (walk/run bike on the pier – all around to be fair to all participants with bike shoes on) and figure out where you finish the bike (bikes are taken from you at the bike finish by a friendly and patient volunteer—what a dirty job.). Following a walk through from the bike finish back to collect your T2 run bag, you head to the changing tent to get into your run gear.

Race day morning, I usually do another walk through after I pump up my tires and stock my bike with fuel (water bottle, Generation UCAN, Hammer Nutrition supplements— "pill bags"—and my "Raw Revolution" real food bars.) I also get my swim gear organized. Then, I find a quiet spot to relax, get my mind right, and do some yoga mobility work until the race director calls us over the loud speaker to enter the ocean.

Reality sets in!

It's game time.

The nerves start to increase, but the challenge for me was always how to stay in a positive mindset and not stress about the swim as my strength was on the bike then be ready for the run. The march of the triathletes into the water made us look like cattle being called to dinner. We enter the timing mats to the swim start. Any Ironman swim start (mass swim start) is always hectic, crowded, and a bit of insanity topped with a dash of anxiety.

The World Championship deep water swim start is even more of a circus since you have 1,600 or more top triathletes from the around the world all ready to compete at once. Swimming 2.4-miles with 1,600 plus people requires a positive mindset and attitude, to say the least. I try to think of the swim as a game, concentrating on which swimmer to be beside in order to get a little draft (less work) and swim faster without exerting any extra energy.

The IM swim start line is also a game of patience as we have to wait so long (feels like we are waiting for an hour) once we are waiting in the deep water start line. Paddle boarders and surfboarders line up to hear the Hawaiian music playing on the speakers. The most important Ironman Triathlon race of the year is beginning. The world's best age group long distance triathletes are going to start the big dance.

The dance starts in the ocean off the swimming pier in Kona. Once we walk in along the small sandy area of "Dig Me" beach, we begin our warm up to swim to the starting area in the deep water. We end up having to tread water for at least fifteen minutes in the Hawaiian ocean swells, trying not to run into the paddle boarders blocking the start line.

It's time… the blow horn goes off earlier for the professional men and the women's groups, (separate starts) then for the age groups making it one mass start in the deep blue ocean waters of Hawaii at 7:00 a.m. sharp.

BOOM!

Once the sound goes off and you hear the planes fly above, we all take off at once. The journey has begun for the day. The kickoff to our long day is to swim 2.4-miles in the Hawaiian blue ocean (while I search for dolphins swimming under us), then bike 112-miles along the lava fields with the trade winds, and finally to run a grueling 26.2-miles along the hot pavement in the afternoon Kona sun, hoping to cross the finish line by sunset.

Ironman can take the professionals under eight hours, but others up to twelve hours with the last finishers having to be done by midnight. That's seventeen hours of entertainment, excitement, and building memories that will last a lifetime.

My best time previous Ironman time was at Ironman Canada in 2012, under 10:22 and my previous best time at Ironman Hawaii was a 10:34, so, of course, I had to set my new goal to be under 10:15 for my Hawaii finishing time in 2012. As you know by now, you should never compare race times on different courses, especially with the unpredictable weather. Just as in life, we need to re-assess our goals if we are in the pursuit of "happiness" by reaching our goal times. Perhaps, we should not depend on finding happiness by finishing a race at a setup and instead simply be happy by finishing a race most people can only dream about entering, never mind completing.

In the 2012 Ironman World Championship race, after coming off of an unreal triathlon season, my race times, when I wanted to be my best, were not what I'd planned for that day with my high personal standards and expectations of myself. However, the weather is out of my control. What is in my control is how I *handle* the emotions, how I react to the weather conditions, and my mindset.

You must remember everyone else on the course is dealing with similar conditions, so you have to let go of any prior goal times and keep re-assessing your race strategy as it is happening. My splits that year were slower than my previous race in Kona and definitely slower than at Ironman Canada, but you can never compare times on different race courses or even the same course with varied weather patterns as Kona.

Although my finishing time and splits were respectable for Ironman Hawaii, but I did not make my dream 10:30 finishing time! We did have a headwind all the way back from the turnaround in Hawi and along the Queen K back into Kona for the transition to the run (T2). I never seem to be satisfied with my accomplishments- I always believed I could do better and be faster!

> Ironman Hawaii 2012 Results:
> **Potts, Deborah, W40-44**
> Overall time 10:58:17/overall 908 and 15th overall in my age group
> Swim: 1:18:34/T1 3:35/Bike 5:42:51/T2 2:25/Run 3:50:54

Why do I set high standards for myself and set goals that challenge my ability and performance?

After seeing my performance gains over the years with my Mark Allen (MA) coaching, the MA Elite Team motivation (everyone was so strong, powerful, and successful on our team), and my strength training work, I believed in my abilities and setting goals is important for me in order to take it (me) to the next level and grow. I strive for optimal health, of course, but who do I try to impress by myself?

No one else but my husband really understood what my race splits were about, plus I never spoke about my races, results, and/or accomplishments to my "non-triathlon" friends and clients. Why bother anyone with my race stories? It was how I rolled at the time, but I do wish now I would have been more proud and grateful for my accomplishments.

Ironman Hawaii 2010 Results:
Potts, Debbie USA W35-39
Overall time 10:34:21/799 overall/11 overall in my age group *(top 11 in the world should be something to be excited about, but not until now)*
Swim: 1:13:21/T1 3:49/Bike 5:29:02/T2 3:05/Run 3:45:06

Personally, Kona is my special place where I feel the energy of the island and its magic every time I arrive on the island. Especially after I'm there for a day or two and I let my guard down to embrace the aloha spirit. I experienced the power of the island god, Madame Pele, my first year training on the course and on race day starting at the Ironman Hawaii World Championship back in 2004. My first few times riding the IM bike course were with a smile on my face and a sense of peace and calmness while I sang my magic Kona bike song all the way along the Queen K Highway with the unpredictable winds that can beat you down and even break you if you let yourself be vulnerable.

I always feel the presence of Madame Pele watching over me and protecting me all the way up to the rolling hills filled with potential harsh side winds that can send your bike sailing into the air, up toward the small town of Hawi. I felt safe as I descended quickly on my bike along the crazy downhill roads from Hawi with the chance again of the battle against the side winds of the beautiful blue ocean. As I make my way back to Kona to the transition area, I would always be singing my magic Kona IM song and praying to feel as if I had the wind at my back, even if it was blowing me sideways or fighting me head on. I would be strong mentally and physically to win the battle of the Kona winds.

Once you get on the run course in an Ironman, you feel as if you are almost near the finish line even though you have 26.2-miles to complete prior to reaching the magical emotional finish line. My strategy in an Ironman is to focus on running one mile at a time with a quick pause and reset at each aid station every mile on the course. At each reset station, I would take a cup of ice and a cup of water to keep from melting and shriveling up on the side of the road on the hot pavement (or jumping in the ocean when we run along Ali'i Drive) in the hot sun.

Another one of my training secrets on race day is to pace myself on the bike by keeping my heart rate aerobic (MAF, which is discussed in The WHOLESTIC Method manual chapter on exercise) and avoid consuming sugar (another topic to get off the blood sugar roller coaster). The trick in an Ironman, especially in Kona, is to leave something in the tank for the run so by being a fat burning machine and metabolically efficient (still burning fat at higher heart rates to avoid early fatigue), I'll have something left in my legs to run 26.2-miles without blowing up as many triathletes do on the run portion of an Ironman because they ride too hard on the bike part. I actually have run faster the last few miles when I head toward town to the amazing finish line chute.

I always have difficulty explaining what the Ironman Hawaii race day experience is about for the athlete and the spectator unless you have been fortunate enough to be at one memorable day as it is thrilling and magical for everyone involved.

The finish line in Ironman Hawaii is one of the most magical and powerful experiences for anyone. Even watching the replay on NBC still gives me goosebumps and puts tears in my eyes. When you turn the corner to the finish chute on Ali'i Drive and run along with all the spectators cheering for you, it sure makes your run faster, especially when they're giving you high fives. You must be getting the mojo from the participants and it works to propel you on.

When I see my magic tree, I know I am almost there. I'm on the last sprint to the finish line, and then I can stop moving and jump in the shower by the beach. The crowd yells your name (it's printed on my race bib), my legs feel suddenly refreshed and temporarily recovered from their exhaustion from an incredibly long day "at the office." You run up the ramp to cross the Ironman Hawaii finish line and go right through the banner. You hear what every triathlete loves to hear... what makes the long challenging and painful day all worth it...

"Debbie... you're an IRONMAN!"

There's no high like the one you feel after crossing that finish line. You have goose bumps from head to toe, your endorphins are on overdrive, your cheeks hurt from smiling so hard, and you've never been more proud of yourself.

Chills on my skin.

Tears in my eyes.

... and, now I want to just take my shoes off.

The finish line experience begins.

But, my race isn't over until I do my customary push-ups – a personal tradition I started after a challenge to do one push-up at the finish line from my trainer friend, Jeff. So, of course, at the finish area of Ironman Hawaii back at the swimming pier where we started less than eleven hours earlier, I drop down and do fifteen push-ups.

Following that, you get your two aides or assistants that come help you as most of us can't walk or move anymore. It's crazy how the body and mind works. I really earned my Ironman Hawaii finishing medal, T-shirt, and swag.

Finally, I get to take a fresh water shower or jump in the ocean after a day of sweat, salt, and sticky beverages all over me. Unfortunately, this is when nausea hits me. My body doesn't know what to do once I reach the finish line at any IM, so I have to keep moving to gradually cool down. I can never eat or drink for hours after I finish. Only pure ginger ale works for me.

It is an Ironman Hawaii tradition to have everyone come out to watch the last hour of the race as the deadline to finish is midnight – a total of seventeen hours. We love to watch the last finishers cross the line in the last hour up to the closing ceremonies at midnight. The Hawaiian closing ceremonies with the fire dance always concludes the event. And, there you have it; another day in history has been completed for the Ironman Hawaii World Championship.

At the end of the long, productive, amazing, hard day, I finally get to go to bed and crash, but my body is always too wired from the physical and mental exhaustion one experiences on any IM race day, especially Kona. I can't fall asleep. The adrenaline and endorphins eventually wear off in a few days, but it takes some playing in the ocean and the beach to complete the amazing week in Kona, Hawaii.

The race is over until next year… hopefully.

Onwards and upwards.

Even though I finished the race season of 2012 on an amazing high, I still asked myself:

Can it be repeated? I can do better next year…

4. The Bus Ride that Changed my World

"Eventually, all the pieces fall into place. Until then, laugh at the confusion, live for the moment, and know that everything happens for a reason."
– Albert Schweitzer

What happens when you feel off balance and not your normal self? We often don't realize not feeling your "normal" isn't actually... normal.

We don't have to feel fat, tired, fatigued and depressed- instead, we can find answers instead of complaining. We need to realize our new "normal" isn't acceptable and long term. Instead of adjusting to the "new" you, we can take action and do something about it (and not blame the aging process.)

There are solutions out there to most of your symptoms that arise, but we have to know where to look and who to talk to get results. Remember to "own your own health" and not settle for less instead of sitting on the sidelines and just adapting to feeling crappy, lazy and fat is how life is going to be from now own. The first step is experiencing a "wake up" call to create that internal alert or set off your alarm system that there is something "off" inside that needs to be attended to immediately. The "mind-body" emergency room to re-adjust your HPA-Axis.

I couldn't pinpoint what exactly was wrong with me until I had a horrible experience that was seriously unlike me. I had a major wake-up call. Unfortunately, my experience was in front of sixty people—peers on a bi-annual Mastermind Retreat.

I am a member of Todd Durkin's Mastermind group (TDMM), a group of health and fitness professionals who all strive to inspire and impact the world. Part of our TDMM mission statement shares:

"We are a tribe of pioneers who collaborate on the most effective ways to shape the fitness industry and improve lives of the people around us."

Todd Durkin is an internationally recognized strength, speed, and conditioning coach, personal trainer, bodyworker, motivational speaker, and author who motivates, educates, and inspires people worldwide. Our Mastermind group (around one hundred people from around the world) meets two times a year for a retreat in order to get live connect time, get creative, act on our intentions and go deep on creating our vision in our business (and life.).

So, when we had our retreat in San Diego in 2013, I was feeling intense or rather tense? I was feeling more serious and emotional than other group event and this wasn't because of our group educational sessions that often require us to focus inward and do a lot of writing. I didn't meet the groups for the morning workout sessions as I had to do my triathlon training scheduled swim workout (in an amazing quiet outdoor pool next door to the hotel) or lunch time as I would only eat low-carb/high-fat food – or after the sessions for happy hour socials as I needed to go for my scheduled training run. I realized I was self-conscious and insecure all weekend. I was not feeling the "normal" happy me. Why was I suddenly feeling so anxious, serious, and uptight around my teammates? What was going on with me? Why did I feel so out of place and uncomfortable around the people who were there to support and lift me up? These were my teammates and family.

Red flag alert that I was unaware of at the time was telling me something was definitely off with me.

Then, my wild girl kicked in and my life-changing evening started. My life, as I knew it, started to unravel. My current way of living life was about to come to a drastic end... my breaking point was during the Saturday evening social event. After each day (Friday and Saturday), we have a special TDMM dinner event somewhere fun to end our weekend.

For this retreat, we stayed in the beautiful Torrey Pines area of the famous golf course overlooking the ocean cliff. Typical me, after a long day in an intense group seminar inside (on a beautiful sunny day) on Saturday, I had to get outside for fresh air and exercise. I only had a short period of time to fit in my run interval workout and dressed for the party. I always know how to cram more into one hour and do more than I should be doing.

I was having so much fun running and being in the California sunshine it was hard to turn around and head back to the hotel to stay on time. I had to rush (red flag alert) to get ready for the bus departure. I, of course, ran longer than I should have and had to hurry to get ready for the party. Rush, rush, rush and still no food and not enough water. My extra few minutes of extra running created a race and rush to get showered, dressed up, and ready for the TDMM evening party event. The teams were to meet around 6:00 p.m. outside the hotel lobby to take a real decked out real party bus (that I only thought college kids or a bachelorette party would use.)

The bus ride from Torrey Pines to the winery up north on the packed California freeways took a lot longer than expected by the organizers planned due to a major accident or construction that had us moving slowly on the freeway. Actually, I had no clue what was going on as I wasn't really conscious. We were on our way to a sit-down dinner reserved for the TDMM group, but we were a bit late. Julie, the organizer for our events, thinks of everyone and every detail. She'd stocked the party bus with snacks and wine for our commute to the winery.

The Party Bus ride experience was my major eye-opening wake-up call and the morning after was the beginning of a new crazy ride starting with one majorly long hangover with a taste of alcohol poisoning. The story I am about to share with you is very unlike me and quite embarrassing. Since I started competing in cycling events, marathons and triathlons in my mid-twenties, I stopped going out Saturday nights to the bars. Instead, I preferred to get a good night sleep and so I could wake up in the morning feeling fresh, prepared and recovered to do a long training bike or run workout with my training partners. Instead of spending an evening out drinking too much- and waking up with a hangover (as I seem to easily get sick from drinking alcohol especially in college), I switched over the years to drinking soda waters with lemon or lime instead of a beer or cocktail to pretend I was drinking. I'd rather feel good the next day to do my triathlon training workout instead of dealing with the toxins from alcohol in my body.

However, this particular time, place, and circumstance seemed that I needed to make an exception to my typical behavior. After feeling uptight and too tense all weekend at our retreat, I thought I would attempt to unwind (by drinking wine) by becoming a relaxed "Fun Debbie." In my effort to lower my guard or the wall I had built up around me, I surrendered to interpreted peer pressure. The outcome wasn't pretty. Debbie drank too much wine too quickly on too empty of a stomach.

I obviously had a very low tolerance for alcohol and wasn't used to drinking anymore. The plastic travel glasses of red wine (I kept getting a refill to let loose and fit in). It was a bit much for pure clean me – and that was only the first half of the ride. I never consciously experienced the second half of the bus ride or the dinner party at the winery.

As it stood, I didn't eat much during the entire Mastermind retreat, partially as I was pretty serious about eating real unprocessed food, low carb, and higher healthy fat so if the food that I would eat wasn't available then I wouldn't eat. I was fueled by coffee and water for the past few days plus my few "acceptable" low-carb/high-fat snacks I purchased at the local Whole Foods (high maintenance me – I know it already). To make a long story short, I never made it off the bus for dinner at the winery that night and I wasn't even aware when we arrived at the location.

As I was trying to relax and let loose with the TDMM crew in the back of the bus (I was sitting in the last seat next to my coach, Larry), I was feeling too uptight and serious that I was irritating myself. The red wine was being served quickly amongst the people I was sitting around (younger guys who drank a lot more frequently than I did.) The alcohol hit me almost instantly (from what I can remember and from what I was told later.) My surroundings became blurry and the room was spinning. It was not a great feeling to add being car sick and claustrophobic in the very last seat of a big bus.

I was told later that I passed out before we arrived at the winery. I am not sure how long I was out, but when I woke up, I was alone on the bus with a few people watching out for me. It felt as if I had been asleep for the entire night. I was completely confused as to where I was and what had happened, but I did realize I was feeling violently ill and had to "continue" the detox process in the back of the bus.

No more details needed...

Well, I did have a few bad flashbacks of being very sick in the tiny bathroom in the back of the bus. Thankfully, we had a bathroom on the bus. When I became somewhat alert, the team was coming back on the bus after the dinner party. Once I was more awake, I panicked and needed off the bus to get fresh air and be sick again. In order to get off the bus as people were coming the other way to get back to their seats, I had to do the "walk of shame" in front of my teammates (most of whom I didn't know well). As I was walking gingerly, I felt dizzy and queasy, basically extremely drunk, poisoned, and starting the detox or begin the hangover process.

Some of my teammates had their own car so, fortunately, I didn't have to get back on the bus in front of the group again and ride back to the hotel. I was like a happy dog hanging its head out of the car window on the drive all the way back to Torrey Pines with the exception of a few stops we had to pull over on the side of the freeway for me to "detox." Eventually, I got to my hotel room and passed out on the bed until the next morning.

Red flags: stress, empty stomach, dehydrated, sugar and not used to drinking alcohol. These five things *do not* mix well, at all. Any type of stimulant will fuel the sympathetic nervous system, which by now you know is the fight or flight emergency build in response system.

Again, this is another source of stressor that we bring in our lives without being aware of the impact the alcohol is creating to our inside health... most people just drink to feel "happy," "calm," and "relaxed," but what else is alcohol do to your body when consumed daily or in excessive? You may not feel any different on the inside over time with excessive sources of external stress as alcohol and sugar, but wait for what may come in your future. The key point is that too much of anything is toxic. Are you getting my point that "stressors" doesn't only come from a bad relationship or sitting in traffic? External and internal sources are all around us- and accumulate.

From my "walk of shame" off the bus to get a ride in front of sixty other Mastermind team members that were mostly new acquaintances, I not only woke up with the worst hangover of my life but also a complete and total embarrassment. As a non-drinking competitive "healthy" pure athlete, wow, did I ever pay the price of trying to "let loose" and take my guard down. I am sure there are better solutions to letting go anxiety than with alcohol. Going overboard cost me more than five days of feeling as if I had alcohol poisoning and more internal damage.

Now, my friends will understand why I am afraid to drink more than two alcoholic drinks to this day. I never want to experience how I felt that Saturday night on the party bus and the day after. That was a nightmare not to replicate. I thought I'd learned my lessons with drinking too much alcohol in my first year of college, but nothing compared to the repercussions from the party bus.

What I learned the night of the party bus ride was not about me trying to be "Fun Cool Debbie" or overindulging on wine, but rather it was a slap in the face provided by my own body or inner self. I clearly did not pay attention to any of the "red flags" that were given to me over the previous months and this was the last and final step to get me to stop continuing down this path of self-destruction. The reality was I was not healthy on the inside; I was destroying myself from the inside out from my busy non-stop lifestyle. The constant busyness, training, and racing was just adding to the accumulation of stressors in my life.

Just as an alcoholics or drug addict slowly kill themselves (liver and kidney failure) from the inside out by over indulging on excessive amounts of drugs, I was overindulging on the busyness of life. My body and mind were finished with me and this weeklong killer hangover was payback.

The sugar and the alcohol in the wine threw me for a loop because of my exhausted adrenal glands. My body was angry at me and let me know in no uncertain terms.

Here is some information on alcohol as it relates to those with adrenal dysfunction from Brandon Derrow of Doctor Wilson's Original Formulations:

> *Alcohol is a special kind of poison for the adrenals that should not be consumed by people suffering from hypoadrenia. Alcohol is a naked carbohydrate in an extremely refined form (more refined than white sugar) that quickly finds its way into the cells of your body, forcing them to make energy at a rapid rate.*
>
> *This sets off the blood sugar roller coaster that uses up a large number of your body's nutrients that are not replaced by the alcoholic beverage. Tintera, in his excellent 1955 article on hypoadrenia, comments on two kinds of alcoholism related to the adrenals. In one, the alcohol craving is driven by the body's desperate need for quick energy that results from weak adrenals.*
>
> *The alcohol temporarily compensates for the signs and symptoms of hypoadrenia, but leads to further adrenal dysfunction after the effects of the alcohol have worn off, thus producing a further need for alcohol. In the other, the person*

becomes hypoadrenic as a result of alcohol consumption.

If, despite these warnings, you are going to consume alcohol, follow these pointers:

1. *Consume it only in small quantities and on a full stomach.*
2. *Have alcohol with meals that are high in fats or oils as the fats and oils help inhibit the absorption of alcohol and moderate its sudden impact on your cells.*

The universe gave me a message that night which I could not ignore: *slow down and stop living each day as another race.* I was fitting in my triathlon training fasted workouts in between full days of intense sessions at the retreat, with limited food options (that met my high maintenance criteria) while doing intermittent fasting to force my body to burn fat for fuel. The fasting was easy for me because I was not full from eating a high fat and lower carbohydrate food plan which resulted in feeling satisfied for hours with no cravings for sugar. I was demanding a lot from my body and mind.

Fasting can elevate cortisol levels and I was doing a lot of fasting these days. One of the effects of the stress hormone cortisol is raising blood sugar in emergencies as hypoglycemia or a threat. So, for someone with blood sugar regulation or adrenal issues, fasting can actually make them worse. When patients try intermittent fasting, their blood sugar control gets worse. Practitioners will see fasting blood sugar readings in the 90s and even low 100s, in spite of the fact that they are eating a low-carb, Paleo-type diet. Ideal blood sugar ranges 70-90 mg/dl- below normal range is hypoglycemia and too high blood sugar is hyperglycemia (more in my The WHOLESTIC Method manual.

A great leader to follow (and learn from) in the functional and integrated medicine field is Chris Kresser. *Chris Kresser, M.S., L.Ac is a globally recognized leader in the fields of ancestral health, Paleo nutrition, and functional and integrative medicine. He is the creator of ChrisKresser.com, one of the top 25 natural health sites in the world, and the author of the New York Times best-seller, Your Personal Paleo Code (published in paperback in December 2014 as The Paleo Cure).*

On Chris Kresser's blog, he talked about blood sugar regulation and cortisol imbalances (adrenal issues like mine) in his "Intermittent fasting, cortisol and blood sugar."

"*From an evolutionary perspective, intermittent fasting was probably the normal state of affairs. There were no grocery stores, restaurants or convenience stores, and food was not nearly as readily available or easy to come by as it is today. Nor were there watches, schedules, lunch breaks or the kind of structure and routine we have in the modern world. This means it's likely that our Paleo ancestors often did go 12-16 hours between meals on a regular basis, and perhaps had full days when they ate lightly or didn't eat at all. So, while I agree that IF is part of our heritage and that it can be helpful in certain situations, I don't believe it's an appropriate strategy for everyone. Why?* **Because fasting can elevate cortisol levels**. *One of the cortisol's effects is it raises blood sugar. So, for someone with blood sugar regulation issues, fasting can actually make them worse.*

I don't think eating every two to three hours is 'normal' from an evolutionary perspective. But, neither is driving in traffic, worrying about your 401k, or staying up until 2:00 a.m.

on Facebook. The Paleo template is there to guide us, but it's not a set of rules to be followed blindly. This should also be a reminder that there's no 'one size fits all' approach when it comes to healthcare. Successful treatment depends on identifying the underlying mechanisms for each individual and addressing them accordingly.

Source: http://tinyurl.com/FastingBloodSugar

The adrenal glands produce hormones that help us balance our blood sugar as well as manage the fluctuations in energy throughout the day. I talk in The WHOLESTIC Method manual frequently about the blood sugar roller coaster—when the blood sugar levels drop—the adrenal glands produce hormones that cause the blood sugar to rise and increases energy.

As you have learned already, the adrenal glands (that sit on top of your kidneys) release the main stress hormones cortisol and DHEA when we are feeling stressed and respond to the perceived emergency situation with our natural "fight or flight" response. We don't have the life necessity or requirements (to stay alive) as our ancestors did to have the ability to be ready to run fast when being chased by a lion or tiger... instead, our society requirements command us to respond to an emergency when we are being chased by life stressors including sources of stress from work, traffic, people and manufactured foods except our stressors are non-stop.

Both stress and adrenal dysfunction can contribute to hypoglycemia (low blood sugar) because of the key roles the adrenal hormones epinephrine, norepinephrine and cortisol play in blood sugar regulation. Stress (and the anticipation of stress) signals the body to raise blood sugar (glucose) levels in order to generate energy to respond to the stress. If the body cannot meet this higher demand for blood glucose, hypoglycemia can result. Stress may also provoke blood sugar swings that can have a cumulative effect on the body's ability to maintain blood sugar balance, and aggravate hypoglycemic symptoms. In fact, some of the symptoms of hypoglycemia, such as irritability and nervousness, may sometimes be the effects of high levels of stress hormones rather than of the low blood sugar itself. During adrenal dysfunction, when adrenal hormone levels are lower, it becomes harder to maintain blood sugar balance, especially in response the increased demand from stress.

Source: http://tinyurl.com/BloodSugarRegulation

If we are constantly under stress, the adrenal glands run out of steam and stop producing sufficient amount of hormones. When our "stress response" system (HPA Axis and hormones) are exhausted, we feel depleted, depressed, and out of balance. By continuing to consume various "stimulants" such as coffee, we are only adding more stress to our already broken body. This would be comparable to filling your gas tank with extra fuel and flooding the engine.

If we continue to put more stress on the stressed adrenal and over tax the messengers (brain: hypothalamus-pituitary gland which controls hormone production), then we eventually break the response system, as I did. I was thriving on adrenaline, caffeine, and the sugar and alcohol from the red wine. These things did a number on my body since key roles of adrenal hormones epinephrine, norepinephrine, and cortisol contributes to blood sugar regulation.

I don't know if this is why I had such intolerance to the alcohol and the aftermath of "the bus ride from hell" as enough to investigate the *why*.

The Blood Sugar Seesaw: How Stress Disrupts the Balance:

Your body and brain depend on balanced levels of blood sugar (glucose) to steadily supply your cells with fuel for energy. Stress normally drives blood sugar up to power a "fight or flight" physical response via the adrenal stress hormone cortisol. Cortisol converts energy stored in your body into glucose so that your blood sugar rises to energize that anticipated surge in activity. As your blood sugar goes up, insulin is secreted by your pancreas to move the glucose from your blood into your cells. This extra glucose is meant to be used up by a strenuous physical response to the stress, which restores blood sugar back to normal. In the prehistoric world, stress typically came from physical threats against which a short burst of activity increased the odds of survival. However, in the modern world stressors are typically ongoing pressures against which physical activity is seldom used or useful. If your life is stressful, especially with a diet high in refined carbohydrates and without regular vigorous exercise, the consequent repeated or chronic blood sugar and insulin elevation you experience can create problems over time that prehistoric humans probably never had to face. When this occurs too frequently, your cells become more resistant to insulin to avoid the toxicity of excess glucose. This can leave too much glucose in your blood and too little in your cells. To maintain balance, your body converts and stores the excess blood sugar as fat – usually around your abdomen.

Source: https://adrenalfatigue.org

You can only push yourself for so many years before you crash like I did in the back of the bus. My "bus ride from hell" wasn't a result of my having too much wine. That was merely the cherry on top of an already accumulated sundae of stressors. Once your adrenal glands have worked overtime for so long (living with the "cruise control" button on all day every day), they stop producing enough of the stress hormones to keep up with our demand -and we end up with a dysfunctional adrenal gland resulting in a downhill spiral from the inside out.

I continue to review my previous life to visualize when I had the red flags of having adrenal dysfunction (high or low cortisol), but I assume that was my "normal" way of living. Evidently, I am not able to ignore this major slap in my face alcohol consumption also increases stress hormones (cortisol specifically) in your body and sadly also increases belly fat that I was also experiencing.

Finally, I heard the message loud and clear—although it took a few days to sink in—that something was seriously wrong on the inside. I needed to take action.

The day after my drunken mess, and disastrous embarrassing night with my peers, I thought I'd be able to continue my normal routine including my training schedule. The morning after, I attempted multiple times to drag myself out of bed to go for my swim in the beautiful outdoor pool next to the hotel then one more run along the cliffs of Torrey Pines and into La Jolla, but I was unsuccessful.

My hotel room (fortunately I didn't have a roommate nor did Neal come with me to the retreat) was spinning or rather my head was spinning… and I felt like a Mack truck had run over me. After a few more to fall back asleep to help the recovery process from my horrific hangover, I finally got myself dressed and out of the hotel room early Sunday morning. I had to get moving as we needed to check out by 12:00 p.m. and I had another meeting to get to in downtown San Diego before my flight back to Seattle that evening.

Once I finally walked cautiously from the hotel to the outdoor lap swimming pool without getting sick (and without seeing too many TDMM members in the hallway), then next step was getting into the pool. Swimming in the fresh air sounded like the perfect solution to my hangover, but swimming freestyle with a dreadful headache and the spins does not work. I don't know if it is possible to swim laps when you are nauseated as you have to position your body supine and attempt to complete a few proper freestyle strokes (or even breaststroke would work) to get to the other end of the pool without sinking (or drowning). Before I knew it, I was back in my hotel room requesting a late checkout. I was back on my bed waiting for nausea to end and the room to stop spinning. There was no way I was going to make it on my long run either. Not a good start to a picturesque Sunday morning.

Needless to say, the rest of my Sunday was a disaster and then the start of my 2013 Ironman training schedule was in question until I had some answers.

A transformation was required if I wanted to return to competing in Ironman, or, more importantly, not have more serious health problems. My major life transformation lesson, awareness, mission, and the journey began that day after the party bus experience.

Gradually, I realized I had a new mission: I needed to start living from the inside out as a The WHOLESTIC Method athlete if I ever wanted to reach my peak performance again in triathlons… and in life. A serious intervention was mandatory in order for me to get this transformation process started to improve the WHOLE me from the inside out.

That first intervention happened in the hotel elevator when my Mastermind teammate, Heather, stepped in the elevator with me. Since I was so embarrassed to see anyone from the Mastermind team after the party bus episode (the passing out for hours, the bathroom and the walk of shame), I felt the need to apologize to everyone who I had contact with on the "morning after" for my extreme behavior. In my mind, my reputation as a top competitive age-group triathlete was tarnished. Instead of "Debbie Diesel" or the "triathlete girl," I would now be labeled as the girl who couldn't hold her alcohol. But, why was I worrying so much about what other people thought of me?

Because we all do on some level.

I'd struggled with confidence and self-esteem through my teenage years and into college. It's bad enough being a teen girl with the traditional angst and emotions, but I was also taller than most other girls. I was always trying to find the *right* group to hang out with in; wanting to be friends with most all groups or be in each clique. Most of my insecurities are to blame for being taller than most boys in school. I never had a boyfriend nor was I invited to a school dance or the prom. Perhaps my childhood tall girl insecurity, low self-esteem, and lack of confidence were based on an athletic image I'd created as an adult.

Let's go back to my conversation with Heather in the elevator. Timing was everything. We learn a valuable life lesson in all life experiences.

I knew Heather to be a student in the Kalish Institute training to become a Kalish Method Practitioner. I had heard about Dr. Dan Kalish and his Kalish Method from listening to a few health and fitness podcasts he'd been interviewed on. The

Kalish Method is "a functional medicine [treatment or medical practice focusing on the body's function and its organs using a system of holistic or alternative medicine], lab-based health approach focused on addressing five common conditions – weight gain, fatigue, depression, female hormones, and digestive problems – through restoring the three main body systems: hormones, digestion, and detoxification," according to Dr. Kalish's website. (You can hear my podcasts with Dr. Dan Kalish on www.thewholeathletepodcast.com.)

After my long-winded apology to my team member Heather for what happened on the party bus, she suggested my reaction to the wine and exertion might point to me having some adrenal issues. The universe (or someone above) was bringing us together for my first step to getting guidance and direction. I guess my obsessive behavior with my food (diets started back in seventh grade.), training, and uptight serious (at the time) personality was obvious to outsiders while my behavior was the standard way of living and operating in daily life.

So, when Heather mentioned the Kalish Institute, I became instantly intrigued and I wanted to know everything immediately as we were talking about my health and well-being and my future as an IM Athlete.

I asked her to provide more specific information on hormone health and adrenals related to my situation based on her observations on my behavior, personality and reaction to alcohol the previous night. I wished she would help save me from whatever was going on inside of me- I wanted her to share all the secret tips that would help me immediately as I was on a schedule. In a few months, I had the half Ironman triathlon (Honu 70.3) in Kona then Ironman Canada in Whistler in the summer. I didn't have time to waste and interrupt my training schedule to impair my performance as I had major goals for this season and personal records to set.

Fortunately, Heather suggested I be her case study for the Kalish Method student program she was doing. Thus was the beginning of my recovery from adrenal dysfunction and the start of the Kalish Method protocol in my life.

Ironically, that Sunday afternoon, after my multiple attempts to get out of bed so I could make a weak effort to swim a lap and then experience the biggest challenge of getting showered, cleaned up, packed, and checked out of my hotel room in time, I also had a major networking meeting scheduled. I had reached out to one of my favorite podcasters, role models and peer, Sean Croxton to have a quick conversation while I was in San Diego for the retreat.

I had admired Sean since he'd spoken at my Todd Durkin Mentorship program in 2010. Sean started the "Underground Wellness Radio" way back in 2008 before podcasting was really known. His podcast was all about real food and functional medicine which always inspired me to learn more about these topics as well as become a practitioner myself (learn more about Sean at www.seancroxton.com.) Sean wrote one of my favorite ebooks, "The Dark Side of Fat Loss," where he termed "JERF" (Just Eat Real Food) and was a pioneer in creating online health summits including one for thyroid health, digestion, and depression. This guy was an inspiration to me as well as many other fitness professionals. If they were ahead of the ball game and listened to his podcast, of course, I wanted to set up a meeting with him at the end of my retreat with one of my other mentors Todd Durkin.

But, why did I have to be having the worst hangover of my life (maybe a worse one in my first year of college but that was years ago.). Another day of embarrassment and walking with my tail between my legs.

I always related to Sean's background as a personal trainer who then became frustrated with trying to help clients lose fat, get healthy, and improve performance with exercise alone.

It was odd timing that the day and uncanny especially since this was right after I'd had my intervention with Heather on the Kalish Institute course. I finally was able to meet Sean in his office while secretly being completely hung over and sick. I could barely make it out of the hotel room to meet Sean in his downtown San Diego office. I was throwing up in the parking lot and then in the running a few times to the bathroom at his office building while I was waiting to chat with him. It isn't easy acting sober when needed. I'm not sure how alcoholics live life this way or does it become their "normal?"

Sean frequently had guests on his show like Dr. Dan Kalish and Paul Chek to discuss hormone imbalances, parasites, leaky gut, gluten intolerance, and more health-related information that was only really known in the "underground" world of health podcasts. The man who inspired me from afar to create my own health and fitness podcast was now seeing me as someone who drank too much or had her own problems. Or, he just didn't notice I was experiencing a major hangover. Maybe he thought I had to go to the bathroom a lot and needed to get out in the sun more as I was super pale.

As I look back, these experiences had to have been on purpose; instrumental life transformational interventions. These "meetings" were more of the process to my new beginning and I was suddenly forced to make a life transformation, such as a butterfly.

> *"A butterfly is a magical symbol of great transformation to come. It is a reminder that our current reality is to be experienced so that we may grow to change for the better. We are to accept and embrace these changes while keeping our faith in the end results."*
> – Unknown

Now, I feel it is my new purpose in my lifetime to share my journey and ongoing transformation as an endurance athlete, trainer, coach, small business owner, and spouse. I am devoted (and obligated) to letting nature take its course as I continually

transforming myself with each new experience and journey. As I began to heal and recover from the aftermath of the party bus ride experience then onto discovering what really was happening on the inside- adrenal dysfunction or HPA Axis dysfunction. The party bus ride was the beginning of a slow eruption from the inside of a volcano…lava gradually pouring from the deep inside.

What that the eruption or is there more to come?

In The WHOLESTIC Method program, I wrote in the manual discussing the eight elements and program workbook to help you create your own personal "roadmap." The process of writing and answering the questions in the program workbook will definitely help you determine not only where you are now but also where you are coming from and where you are headed.

The questions I include in the workbook will help you dig deeper into your past and current habits (and mindset). With this information, we can work together to create a new plan, create new habits and create a new roadmap to improve the WHOLE you with The WHOLESTIC Method as I have over the years.

Together, we can get to the root cause of your fatigue symptoms, ask for the right help, and then determine the best healing pathway and WHOLESTIC program specifically for you.

When we have sudden weight gain, new rapid belly fat, brain fog, bloating, gas, depression, mood swings, and more symptoms, we can make lifestyle adjustments to create improvements from the inside out but we need to find the right type of coaching, support, and guidance (as well as lab tests; more lately). You can feel your best again and not blame everything on the aging process.

We have to work on improving the WHOLE you from the inside out first.

Everything Happens for a Reason

5

"This is the beginning of anything you want."
— Dr. Dan Kalish

When I ran into Heather in the elevator after my party bus incident, I knew we the meeting happened for a reason. When I started to be the Kalish Method case study for her in May 2013, I felt my roadmap was being created and my new journey was starting on that morning after the experience. We had a plan of attack and I was motivated to get some answers and fast results! The first step in this endeavor was taking various lab tests.

Heather mailed the kits Dr. Kalish recommends for adrenal dysfunction to me and I would test my saliva, poop, blood, and pee. Once the lab tests were finalized, we reviewed the results. Heather gave me the Kalish Method treatment plan to follow which included supplements, nutrition, and suggestions for lifestyle changes. The food part was the easiest for me as I was already following a real food plan including low-carb/high-fat focused primal Paleo program. I was missing one area in my food plan: no dairy. Moving forward, I had to be strict on eliminating my commercial dairy intake of cream and cheese.

The first round of the recommended lab tests was to determine my cortisol, DHEA, and melatonin levels. Surprise, the saliva lab test results proved I was in what they predicted already: Stage Three Adrenal dysfunction. This is when the cortisol levels are extremely low and the DHEA hormones are low, as well. Next step? How do we get the cortisol and DHEA levels to be in the ideal "happy" range? Lifestyle changes and supplements were ordered.

Over the next few months, I completed very detailed lab tests and then re-tested again in six months (I still keep re-testing to stay on track and not to regress). The treatment plan and lab tests added up financially, but they were a necessity to determine the root cause of what was ailing me since traditional medical doctors didn't run these specific lab tests, especially the gut bacteria and parasite labs.

As I've explained, our body's adrenal glands produce hormones, but so does stress. When we have too much stress, our body functions suffer and we get depleted overall, which brings about things such as depression, fatigue, blood sugar imbalance, etc. If we continue to live with too much stress in any form, our hormone levels drop and lead to burnout. Ideally, our cortisol levels fluctuate throughout the day, but the levels should be higher in the early morning and lower in the evening.

The adrenal glands produce the hormone DHEA and cortisol based on when the brain processes signals of emergency then the pituitary glands secretes adrenocorticotropic hormone (ACTH) as well as secreting cortisol and adrenaline. A little cortisol in the right doses is ideal, but too much cortisol is not good. (I'll discuss this later on.) Too much cortisol lowers our serotonin (neurotransmitters - nature's own appetite suppressant), raises our catecholamine (dopamine and norepinephrine), damages the hippocampus (damages memory and focus) and depletes the sex hormones (www.kalishinstitute.com).

When you learn more about hormone balance and the role of cholesterol with Pregnenolone (the mother of the hormone chart), you will understand cholesterol doesn't deserve the bad rap it has gained over the years. We need it. I continue to share with clients, write blogs, and do podcasts on the elements included in The WHOLESTIC Method including stress, sleep, digestion, and happiness, but even more so lately, I've given information on the myths of cholesterol, saturated fats, and blood sugar instability. I dive into stress and hormones more in The WHOLESTIC Method manual.

We need to learn about "Pregnenolone Steal" and what happens to your other hormones function when one hormone is taken away to rescue another one. When your adrenals are overused and worn out and you don't have enough cortisol to deal with stress, your Pregnenolone hormone saves the day (temporarily) to help progesterone and cortisol continue on with their jobs. I won't go too deep into the hormones and functions as I can refer you to dozens of other resources to learn more from experts.

The Kalish Method made sense to me as a trainer, coach, and athlete with fatigue, weight gain, depression, gut health issues, and more internal problems. The recovery or healing process isn't easy or quick and will take a lot of work on your part.

I was always searching for the quick treatment plan. I believed there must be some supplement I could take that would be my "magic potion" and cure me overnight. I expected I would wake up in a few days or, even a week, feeling strong, lean, and energetic again. The Kalish Method system includes specific lab tests and supplements that do not heal you completely. There is another important essential element for repairing the internal damage created by excessive stress.

The other half of the Kalish Method treatment plan requires you to make specific transformational lifestyle and mindset shifts in order to heal your adrenals, digestive system, detoxification pathways, and balance your hormones. Taking supplements three times a day wasn't the only solution.

Of course, if you are a Typo A personality like me, you will understand my continued search for another solution- even though the answers were generally the same. Slow down and rest more. Even though I was following The Kalish Method protocol in an effort to get healthy and get back to the best me I could be, I continued to research other treatment plans. I was not satisfied with following just one method to heal, treat, and recover from adrenal dysfunction. I wanted to be fixed or healed immediately, so I looked for the "fast track" adrenal support program. My search for a quick solution led me to many other functional medicine practitioners, naturopaths, and doctors.

What was I really searching for?

Did I honestly think I'd find someone who could give me a shot so I could train and race again? Or, a magic elixir so I could automatically drop this extra thirty pounds of body fat? Oh, if some practitioner could simply help me sleep through the night.

The reality was the answer was *inside of me*.

I didn't understand at the time how crazy a schedule I had kept over the last five to ten years. The hours in the fitness industry are crazy then add training for long distance endurance events plus becoming a small business owner. The truth hurts; I wasn't going to recover or be fixed in one month.

All the lab tests and supplements from my Kalish Method testing were similar to various naturopaths and functional medicine doctors in the Seattle area. The difference was I needed to take responsibility for my required lifestyle changes. I absolutely *had* to slow down and stop trying to do so much at once.

How much did I need to slow down?

I thought I was cutting down on training and doing less work each day, but was that enough? What was my speed limit each day? Did I have enough speed bumps placed in my day to catch myself from doing too much and force me to slow down?

I was the one who was self-sabotaging my body from healing. I continued stressing myself out by wondering why this happened to me. Yet, I continued to question…

Why did I deserve to be sidelined from life when I thought I was "the picture of health" and had just come off of my best triathlon race season in my career?

How could someone appear to be fit and strong on the outside, yet be a mess on the inside for so long without really feeling the changes? I wasn't really aware of the gradual breakdown and red flags until I had to stop on my bike ride that one Saturday morning ride when I noticed excess fat deposits on my athletic body. A big slap in my face was required to get to that morning in the elevator with Heather and start my quest for healing.

The answer was clear, all the tests said so.

The reason I'd exhausted my adrenal glands and created a domino effect of problems in the rest of the body was because I ignored the red flags my body was sharing with me—screaming out, in fact.

Over the few years of my recovery from adrenal dysfunction, I often gave up hope that I would ever see a return to the healthy body I'd known before. I wasn't getting the help and guidance I needed, so I continued to get frustrated, angry, and negative. Instead of being discouraged, I constantly reminded myself that I needed to look for the gifts and knowledge available to me from this journey and what "area of opportunity" did I need to create change and growth in.

My personal training client, Clayton, always has that gift of looking at each setback as an opportunity to grow. So true. I didn't need to strive to return the old version of myself; rather, I must get back to a new and improved version of myself as I continue to go through this transformation process, like a caterpillar changing into a beautiful butterfly.

If you are experiencing the same challenges and symptoms, there is a way out. You don't need to give up the hope of being healthy. There is a solution—and not the "I'm getting older" excuse—to feeling fat, fatigued, and depressed.

This is why I was happy to find The Kalish Method to help me get back on the right path. It might not be the best for everyone, but I want to share more details in order to showcase the effects it had on me personally. Hopefully, you can take away helpful information from this, as well.

I wrote a blog post in 2013 as I was dealing with the adrenal dysfunction that describes more about the Kalish Method. Read my blog post at:

http://tinyurl.com/PottsRecovery

Prior to my personal breakdown, I had listened to a few interviews on Sean Croxten's podcast called "Underground Wellness" with Dr. Dan Kalish. I thought they were talking about me. Quickly, I had scheduled interviews with Dr. Dan Kalish for my podcast for endurance athletes with adrenal issues (find in the archives on the website for FIT FAT FAST podcast). In the interviews, Dr. Kalish explained his Kalish Method in more detail. He knew the traditional medical system wasn't able to help treat patients with these various symptoms and reclaim their health. Dr. Kalish discovered in his practice a variety of problems occur at almost the same frequency with almost the same predictable patterns. They are:

The Kalish Method's Big Five:
1. Gaining Fat
2. Fatigue
3. Depression
4. Female hormonal issue
5. Gastrointestinal problems... the gut

When our adrenals become fatigued (Stage One and Stage Two), we have high cortisol. Cortisol is "glucocorticoids" which stabilize the body's blood sugar. When our adrenals become exhausted (stage three), our cortisol levels decrease too low and then we have all systems failure or crash. When we experience chronic stress for an extended period of time, we eventually burn out the adrenals. No more cortisol can be produced since, in stage three, we now have low cortisol and low DHEA hormone levels. You need to make sure you get tested if you have many of the adrenal dysfunction symptoms.

Maybe you crave more sweets and carbs? What happens if we don't produce cortisol? If we are not able to stabilize the blood sugar levels in our body, then we risk damaging the fat-burning metabolism system because it's regulated by cortisol. If our body's digestive system is compromised, we are not absorbing the nutrients from the food we eat, which is a symptom of gut issues. Often, we end up overeating until we feel full which could point to another problem: leptin resistance.

The inability to burn fat while still consuming carbs/sugar can lead to digestion-related issues. Don't eat gluten or soy-based foods; vegetables are where you should get your carbs. This is best achieved through a primal Paleo food plan focusing on low carb/higher fat/moderate protein.

The gut may not be working properly if there are signs of bacterial infection such as yeast overgrowth, gut bugs, and/or fungal overgrowth. Also, we probably have toxins in the body. If the detox pathways are not functioning, then toxins are spreading throughout our body without an escape method. We retain fluids (inflammation) to help buffer the toxins and store fat because we need it for the excess toxins.

The domino effect… if one goes, they all go…
1. Adrenal System
2. Detox System
3. Digestive System

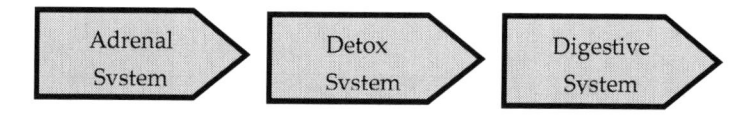

Adrenal System → Detox System → Digestive System

We store excess belly fat due to hormone balancing issues. Eventually, when we do heal the adrenal glands, we can finally burn fat again. Ask your Functional Medicine trained practitioner for natural supplements that work for your needs.

One of the most challenging lifestyle changes I had to make immediately was to stop training long hours and to keep my workout under forty minutes per day to avoid raising my cortisol. Mentally, this was tough for me to do; but physically, I didn't have any other option. My body didn't *want* to train. I was unable to go for a bike ride or a run without having to slow down to walk or even stop altogether.

Here are the other recommendations from The Kalish Method Wellness Program specifically for my use, but they can serve as a guide for you, as well:

1. Gluten-free diet with minimal processed/starchy carbs – do this for sixty days, then reevaluate
2. Eat breakfast within an hour of waking and eat every three to four hours (include protein or no-carb fat)
3. No sugar at all, including reduced sugar from fruit
4. Get to bed by 9:00 p.m. (seven to nine hours of sleep per night) or 8:00 p.m. for my schedule
5. Consider passing on triathlons for a year and focus on strength training, Pilates, and yoga.
6. Keep cardio workouts to forty minutes or less.
7. Get help to reduce emotional stress.

These are the highlights from one of my podcast interviews with Dr. Kalish where he talks more about the effects of excessive athletic training on the body:

- When we do a lot of endurance exercise we put the body in a catabolic state and break down when the body makes stress hormones as cortisol (from cortex).
- When an excessive amount of cortisol is produced from excessive cardio exercise, then we start to break down lean muscle mass.
- We destroy the stomach wall lining and the immune system takes a hit.
- How do we balance catabolic exercise with anabolic exercise? Internally generated hormones.

- It is a domino effect when the cortisol levels are high and the adrenals get exhausted.
- How do we change our training schedule to avoid fatigue and exhaustion? Listen to our past podcasts with Ronda from Sweet Beat on measuring heart rate variability to monitor stress and recovery from workouts.
- When we do cardio for over twenty to thirty minutes then the stress hormone cortisol levels are increased and they can block the conversion of T4 to T3 to disrupt the thyroid gland function.
- Excessive stress depletes the sex hormones as estrogen, progesterone, DHEA, and Pregnenolone.
- When do you take a rest day? More rest days in between exercise sessions and implement strength training sessions the alternate days. What does REST mean to you? I am just learning about what REST is supposed to feel like!
- Most all endurance athletes-triathletes are overtraining and losing muscle mass from over training (related to cortisol). Implement more rest days to get stronger and faster. Less is really more as we age and we get smarter with our training.
- Use strength training to keep tissues and ligaments strong.
- Too much stress will impact the gut wall lining... you may shred the gut wall lining which will cause you to lose

absorption of nutrients. This then results in leaky gut issues as well as a deficiency in Glutamine.
- Return to improved performance levels and reverse the aging process by restoring the hormonal systems imbalance from chronic stress with the Kalish Method system.

Learn more about The Kalish Method and the http://kalishwellness.com.

In order to reclaim my health, I needed to cut out my long workouts to be under forty minutes and add more nature walks. Also, I started to pay attention to my reaction in situations such as driving my car or rushing from masters swim back to my fitness studio to meet a client.

In the past, I never noticed my reaction to stressful events or my lack of patience. I discovered I really needed to reprogram my reactions and relearn how to manage various forms of stress I wasn't aware of in my life. My packed days of going from clients to computer work to masters swim to home for my bike ride and then back to work had to change immediately were over.

For someone like me and all I had accomplished, you can imagine how difficult change would be. My weekends for years included every Saturday Bellevue Club Masters Swim workout at 7:00 a.m. to 8:30 a.m., then home to go on a long bike ride from three to seven hours, depending on the time of year, then maybe a short run. Sundays were spent going for a long run two to three hours in Seattle's Madison Park. Triathlon training was just a way of life… and still is today. I swim, bike, and run four times a week, plus I do yoga and strength training. This had been my routine since 2001. And, it was my reputation.

Even my teammates in my Todd Durkin Mastermind group nicknamed me "Debbie Diesel" during our very first retreat. I would skip lunch so I could get my swim workout in before the second half of our meeting day. I was focused, committed, motivated, and dedicated to my training and racing plan. Maybe a bit obsessed? I think of being too intense as really being too tense... not always a positive attribute and a characteristic to brag about. I was more embarrassed about people asking about my next race and calling me "Debbie Diesel." I obviously had a reputation of racing and competing at a top level. Was that a good thing, though?

How much is too much drive and motivation? When does training become overtraining? The big question over my recovery period was to determine if chronic cardio or endurance training (two hours or longer) exercise is actually healthy for us.

The last few years, I have had to dig deep and redefine what is being healthy and athletic.

Is training for an Ironman a good choice in relation to our health and longevity?

Probably not.

Is it a good way to lose weight?

Probably not.

Is it rewarding and exciting?

Definitely, for me, it was at one point in my life.

And now? Hmmm.

Not sure yet.

As I've mentioned, I feel my purpose in life now is to share my story with athletes of all levels and help them becomes a WHOLE Athlete (check out my podcast, The WHOLE Athlete, on iTunes, Stitcher Radio, or on my website at: www.thewholeathletepodcast.com.)

What is the progression of healing the adrenals and reclaiming our health again?

Let's go a little deeper into what is involved in treating the adrenals or rather the HPA Axis, or rather, my long healing or recovery treatment plan that still continues…

Running from a Lion   6

"Life is not a race, but indeed a journey. Be honest. Work Hard. Be choosy. Say 'thank you,' 'I love you' and 'great job' to someone each day. Take time for prayer. Be thankful. Love your life and what you've been given, it is not accidental. Search for your purpose and do it as best you can. Dreaming does matter. It allows you to become that which you aspire to be. Laugh often. Appreciate the little things in life and enjoy them. Some of the best things really are free. Do not worry. Forgive, if frees the soul. Take time for yourself. Plan for longevity. Recognize the special people you've been blessed to know. Live for today, enjoy the moment."
– Bonnie Mohr

The body's stress control center headquarters—the adrenal glands—release the hormone cortisol in response to stress. If these glands become overworked, fatigued, or exhausted from too much overstimulation due to participating in a daily race, it results in what is termed Adrenal dysfunction.

Adrenal dysfunction is the simplified term for HPA Axis Dysregulation, but it is not recognized by the conventional medical community as a distinct syndrome; however, that doesn't make the problem any less real to those experiencing it.

Whether we choose to live life in the daily human rat race or as an Ironman Triathlon, the end result over time is a breakdown of our hormonal stress response system.

We all have stress, but some people manage it better than others. The source of chronic stress can vary from:

- The frequency and duration of endurance or cardio exercise ("chronic cardio").
- What type of foods you are eating—processed, manufactured, sugar-filled foods we think are "healthy" and good choices, but really aren't.
- Work stress—boss, co-workers, hours, deadlines, and/or workload.
- Daily nerve-racking situations such as computer issues, cell phone distractions, commuting (whether it be in the car or on public transportation), or simply an overscheduled day.
- Toxic or challenging relationships: spouse/significant other, kids, other family members, friends, or the colleagues.
- Stomach infections from leaky gut (bloating, gas, cramps, aches, pains, etc.), parasites, or fungal infection.
- Too many wellness "withdrawals" and not nearly enough "deposits."

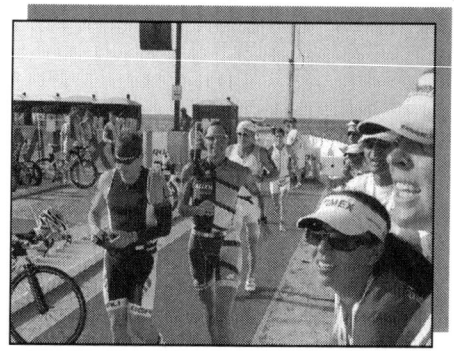

There are many symptoms of adrenal dysfunction, as well as treatment programs that are beyond the scope of this book. I am not a naturopath or functional medicine doctor, but I can share helpful information based on my journey, as well as from my experience and training as a coach and athlete. I am able to refer you to a qualified practitioner who specializes in working with individuals like me who can help you get started with a free consultation and then set you up with a specific treatment plan based on your symptoms, lab tests, and lifestyle improvements.

What is your "area of opportunity?"

What is the one thing you can control and improve today?

> Set up a consultation with Dr. Dan Kalish or one of his practitioners or simply get more information on The Kalish Method at: http://kalishwellness.com/methodology.
>
> Also, check out:
> Christopher Kelly - www.nourishbalancethrive.com
> Dr. Michael Lam - www.drlam.com

Here are some common symptoms of adrenal dysfunction:

- Chronic fatigue or constantly feeling tired
- Belly fat and sudden weight gain Sugar cravings and salty food cravings
- Hormone imbalance and low thyroid symptoms
- Skin issues as rashes, psoriasis or eczema
- Difficulty focusing, memory issues- brain fog, confusion
- Trouble completing tasks and focusing
- Anxiety and emotional instability
- Moodiness, irritability, negative attitude
- Depression and excessive emotions
- New sensitivities and reactions to specific foods

Constant high-stress levels can trigger a domino effect on the internal hormonal systems and lead to many other health issues. According to Janet McGill, MD and hormone specialists from Washington University in St. Louis, fatigue can lead to or be a sign of:

- ✓ Anemia
- ✓ Arthritis
- ✓ Diabetes
- ✓ Heart Failure

According to Robert Vigersky, MD and past president of the Endocrine Society, he confirms that fatigue is due in part to very common problems such as:

- ✓ Stress in the home or workplace
- ✓ Poor dietary habits
- ✓ Poor sleep habits
- ✓ Depression

I can confirm all the above because this is what happened to me in 2013. Personally, I have dealt with the treatment plan for leaky gut symptoms, skin rash, Blasto gut bacterial infection, low immune system, food sensitivities, weight gain, emotional breakdowns, mood swings, constant fatigue, trouble sleeping, and more issues including low thyroid or hypothyroid levels, hormonal imbalance, and disproportional levels of everything in my lab tests.

So many of us live each day without any clue that these multiple health problems are red flags related to our chronic stress because we don't actually think we *are* stressed. We think stress is normal or everyone has it and deals with it. That's simply the way of our society, right? As I said, over time, adrenal stress leads to an internal hormonal crash, including your digestive system, liver detox pathways, and more.

We really don't win anything at the "finish line" by living life as a daily race every day. Are we able to re-learn how to exist in the present by disconnecting and enjoy the moment? Live today in the present and treat it as it is a gift as we never know what tomorrow brings. Avoid getting caught up in our excessive non-stop fast paced life.

Why do we strive to race through the day as if reaching bedtime if our new finish line each day? We have to learn how to pace ourselves by placing our own life "speed bumps" in throughout our day to force us to slow down and pause for a moment. Life is a gift. Let's try to make an effort to stop, re-assess your life goals, improve our daily schedule, re-arrange our priorities, and notice how we feel from the inside out.

Can you learn how to pace yourself differently? If we could begin by realizing we all have a choice of how to live the life we have been given, the results may be different and even more sensational than our current life.

Life is a journey to enjoy, savor, and appreciate.

It's not a race.

If we can gain the tools (The WHOLESTIC Method) to own our health, we can avoid being side struck by the "chronic stress red flags" I share throughout my story. We neglect to pay attention to our own feelings, emotions and body's feedback loop as our body is very intelligent and is supposed to be self-regulating our automatic functions. Instead, we neglect our very own body's way of communicating for help and waving the surrender flag... for some reason, we don't have respect for our own body that we live in.

Remember, the adrenal glands are the main stress control system in the body. Once the brain (hypothalamus) interprets a "threat" and tells the pituitary gland (controls hormone production) to have the adrenal glands respond to the stress by releasing stress hormones as cortisol. I think of stress response system similar to how a house is burning down, then the Emergency Response System (EMS) or 911 is contacted to then sets in motion the response team as the fire department team to come put out the fire. Repeated dependence on the stress response system will deplete and dysregulate the "HPA Axis" and adrenal hormones as cortisol and adrenaline.

As we continue to wear out, exhaust, and break down the function of our adrenals, we weaken the glands. The repeated "crashes" will progressively move us to the next stage of adrenal dysfunction as Dr. Lam focuses on in his practice. As I discovered, exhaustion of the adrenals creates what I term the domino effect internally since multiple organ systems become "systematically decompensated concurrently," according to Dr. Lam.

I agree, as I experienced (and still do) most internal health programs once I hit the "stage three" point of adrenal dysfunction. You name it, I had it. Dysfunction in one system always affects the other parts of the endocrine system. Dr. Lam has found that "the adverse feedback loop creates a vicious cycle of cascading decompensating, involving multiple organ systems at the same time." Dr. Lam continues to share the typical female case involves symptoms of under-active thyroid (me still today), unbalanced ovarian hormones (I never could get pregnant) and obviously low thyroid function.

Source: http://tinyurl.com/LamArticle

If our chronic stress exceeds what is a "normal" amount (and necessary) for our built-in stress response team to respond to daily. The adrenal glands lose their effectiveness and ability to respond to the chronic stressor from life that we are continually exposed to daily. Stressors come in different forms as we keep going over emotional, physical, mental and environmental. (If I keep repeating myself, it's because I want this information to get into your head.)

More specific example includes:

- Anger
- Chronic illness
- Depression
- Surgery
- Excessive intake of sugar
- Over exercising
- Sleep deprivation
- Chronic or acute infections – example gut infections as H. Pylori, Giardia, SIBO and even root canal repair.

I share my red flags and symptoms through this story but some major red flags I see with many clients each day include: most people have no clue they have adrenal issues and struggle to lose weight or get healthy by cutting calories and exercising more. That is not The WHOLESTIC Method approach we take to burn fat, optimize our health, and improve performance.

Let's touch on some of the adrenal dysfunction red flags your body is telling you something is off or overworked on the inside out:

- Gain weight easily and inability to lose weight – especially belly fat around the waistline
- Reduced sex drive, lack of interest, mood, and energy
- Lower immune system – frequent bouts of flu and other respiratory diseases that last longer than usual (I never get sick, but then I would get sick each winter for weeks)
- Inability to deal with stressful situations without feeling anxious, short temper, impatient and emotional (try fixing a flat tire on your bike with people waiting and watching you)
- Being light headed when rising from a prone position (on your back –face up)
- Brain fog and memory issues- difficulty remembering something you just thought of or a name (me all the time)
- Random unknown chronic pain for no specific reason
- Feeling refreshed if takes a vacation (Hawaii for me.)
- Low energy in mid-afternoon (nap time)
- Over dependence on caffeinated beverages, as coffee, to get through the day
- Craving salty and fatty foods- overeating
- Food sensitivities- reaction to various foods that never were a problem
- Low blood sugar or hypoglycemia (blood sugar roller coaster)
- Hormonal imbalance (irregular menstrual cycle)
- Depression over odd things
- Inability to sleep through the night/problems getting back to sleep
- Lack of energy/strength while biking, running, etc.
- Days to recover from simple workouts

Do you find yourself suddenly getting more agitated, short-tempered, and irritable with co-workers, friends, and family, or just in life experiences in general? Perhaps you are feeling more sensitive and emotional each day and find yourself crying for no reason. Is your memory becoming worse, but you blame it on the aging process? One of my personal pet peeves is using aging as an excuse to most changes in our health and performance.

These are what we call "red flags" and symptoms that your stress response system is overtaxed and your new "normal" does not have to become tolerable. Feeling fat, tired, depressed is *not* necessarily a part of "getting older" and our aging process. Personally, I don't like it when people use their aging as an excuse for slowing down or brain fog memory. Yes, it is a fact. We do age up each year, but we don't have to "become old" or feel older if we don't want to; it's our mindset and our attitude toward life. We can approach a new year in life as a new opportunity to grow and transform and strive to age gracefully and slow down the aging process by accepting we have a choice how we want to live our one life that we are given. Own your own health.

There is a light at the end of the tunnel, but we need the right type of light to show us to the other side. We can find the right solutions to our symptoms by finding the right guidance and plan.

"We delight in the beauty of the butterfly, but rarely admit the changes it has gone through to achieve that beauty."
– Maya Angelou

If you dig deeper with a qualified team of experienced experts including a certified health lifestyle coach, nutritional therapist (as myself) and find the best match of a functional medicine doctor who specializes in HPA Axis dysregulation and hormone imbalance in order to get to your "why," then over time, you can find the root cause(s) to your stressors.

Next, you begin your new journey of healing your adrenals, managing stress, and changing your lifestyle habits.

There is a treatment plan for adrenal dysfunction that doesn't involve a prescription drug. Most doctors are not trained in combining functional medicine where they treat the root cause rather than the symptom. Next, we need specific, functional labs tests to get to the root cause of why we don't feel energetic, why we are depressed, and why we are gaining belly fat. We need to get the correct lab testing (saliva, blood, stool and urine) to get some data including hormones levels tested as cortisol, DHEA, melatonin, Pregnenolone, testosterone and more.

Once we begin to figure out why we are stressed out (multiple sources and reasons), create a roadmap and start to focus on improving our lifestyle habits. Our game plan should include techniques and new habits (adding new "speed bumps" into our day) to teach us how to slow down, unplug and breathe more frequently.

You don't have to be a competitive Ironman triathlete or someone who works sixty hours a week on Wall Street to get hit with adrenal issues. It does not discriminate and affects people at all ages, all walks of life, males and females alike. The key is to diagnose it and make substantial changes in your life. We all experience daily stressors, but it depends on how we deal with the "threats" and how we respond to the situation.

I've touched upon a few of my first noticeable "red flags" already as when I felt like I went to bed as a lean, strong, and fit athlete then woke up the next day with the loss of muscle mass and excess of fat spread all over my body, especially my midsection.

When we try to cram even more activities, commitments, and responsibilities into an already full day, the end result is creating another source of stress for our body (brain) to respond to frequently. The frequent stress response leads to chronic stress response if we don't change our ways. In my situation, I was trying to fit in a competitive Ironman triathlon training schedule each week plus strength training, yoga, and Pilates in an already full schedule of owning my own fitness studio, training clients, coaching clients and teaching group exercise sessions (more exercise that "didn't count as a workout.")

Your signs and symptoms might be similar or may be totally different than my own, but you can fill in your own triggers and identify what sets off your stress response system regularly or constantly. The major challenge is to be in tune with yourself and learn how to hear (and feel) what your body is telling you.

My self-esteem and confidence changed, as well. I was embarrassed about the way I looked to others, especially my clients and fellow athletes. I felt as if people were staring at me with puzzled expressions, judging me while they pondered how could the successful triathlete and trainer let herself get so fat and out of shape so quickly? I assumed people were whispering and talking behind my back… and rumors were going around saying, "She probably got lazy and started eating junk food." My self-confidence was soaring downhill at the same time my weight was climbing sky high and my workout performance was swirling down the drain... and then the depression escalated, as well.

To this day, I continue to work on transforming myself from the inside out by changing my habits as increasing my "transition time" between clients, workouts, admin work, and meetings. I continue to **focus** on being present instead of constantly multitasking, the mind always turned "on," and then always feeling rushed to get to the next event or task. Examples of my "rushing" through daily activities: back to back scheduled appointments, finished my workout, getting ready and even I'm eating). I seem to love cramming more in per hour. Someone who used to be a sign of success and being a "winner" who is the first one done?

Life was always a race to the finish line. From my experience and a new journey to find myself, I have gained awareness of how not only how I operate, but how our society thrives each day. Additionally, I've observed habits of clients, friends, and strangers on how we flourish on living in the fast "express lane" of life on "cruise control"—living at full throttle from when our feet hit the floor in the morning until we crash at night.

That was me... plain and simple.

It's what I was all about and how I'd always been.

Until... adrenal dysfunction.

Let's talk about that.

What is Adrenal Dysfunction? 7

"Sometimes the bad things that happen in our lives put us directly on the path to the best things that will ever happen to us."
- Unknown

You can call it adrenal dysfunction, non-Addison's disease, adrenal apathy, HPA Axis dysfunction or just keep it easy and go with chronic fatigue syndrome. It's all the same in my eyes. It's the result of living life each day as a race and it will take a toll on your body and mind. Maybe we call it "chronic stress disease," but it does exist and is a growing concern of mine based on my societal observations.

What is adrenal dysfunction or adrenal exhaustion as it is often unknown or familiar in the traditional medical community? Adrenal dysfunction is not a medically recognized syndrome, so there is no research to be had on it. What is more recognized in the functional medicine world is the result over time of "living each day as a race" and how our health is related to the dysfunction of our hypothalamus-pituitary-adrenal gland axis (HPA axis), which is the communication system between the command center—the brain—and the hormone release centers which have gone haywire.

"Adrenal dysfunction is a collection of signs and symptoms, known as a syndrome that results when the adrenal glands function below the necessary level. Most commonly associated with intense or prolonged stress, it can also arise during or after acute or chronic infections, especially

respiratory infections such as influenza, bronchitis or pneumonia.

As the name suggests, its paramount symptom is fatigue that is not relieved by sleep, but it is not a readily-identifiable entity like measles or a growth on the end of your finger. You may look and act relatively normal with adrenal dysfunction and may not have any obvious signs of physical illness, yet you live with a general sense of unwellness, tiredness, or 'gray' feelings. People experiencing adrenal dysfunction often have to use coffee, colas, and other stimulants to get going in the morning and to prop themselves up during the day.

This syndrome has been known by many other names throughout the past century, such as non-Addison's hypoadrenia, sub-clinical hypoadrenia, neurasthenia, adrenal neurasthenia, adrenal apathy, and adrenal dysfunction. Although it affects millions of people in the U.S. and around the world, conventional medicine does not yet recognize it as a distinct syndrome."

Source: http://tinyurl.com/SignsofAD

Adrenal dysfunction or hypoadrenia are terms used in alternative medicine to describe the unscientific belief that the adrenal glands are exhausted and unable to produce adequate quantities of hormones, primarily the glucocorticoid cortisol, due to chronic stress or infections. Adrenal dysfunction should not be confused with recognized forms of adrenal dysfunction such as adrenal insufficiency or Addison's Disease.

If we ask those medical practitioners that ventured outside of following the symptom-based thinking of traditional medicine practice, then we find various definitions based on what I call "thinking outside of the box" and finally looking at getting to the root cause.

Three parts that work together to regulate functions such as stress response, mood, digestion, immune system, libido, metabolism and energy levels. Before understanding how to fix your Hypothalamic–pituitary–adrenal axis (HPA axis), it's important to understand how the axis works in the first place.

> *"Adrenal dysfunction can wreak havoc with your life. In the more serious cases, the activity of the adrenal glands is so diminished that you may have difficulty getting out of bed for more than a few hours per day. With each increment of reduction in adrenal function, every organ and system in your body are more profoundly affected. Changes occur in your carbohydrate, protein, and fat metabolism, fluid and electrolyte balance, heart and cardiovascular system, and even sex drive. Many other alterations take place at the biochemical and cellular levels in response to and to compensate for the decrease in adrenal hormones that occurs with adrenal dysfunction. Your body does its best to make up for under-functioning adrenal glands, but it does so at a price. Hypothalamic–pituitary–adrenal axis."*
>
> Source: Wikipedia

HPA Axis = the HPA axis includes three specific parts of your body:

1) The hypothalamus (part of your forebrain);
2) The pituitary gland (just below the hypothalamus);
3) The adrenal glands (at the top of the kidneys).

Source: http://tinyurl.com/BenGreenfieldFitness

The HPA axis communicates to three endocrine glands - the hypothalamus, pituitary gland (located below the hypothalamus) and the adrenal gland (top of the kidneys). These organs control our reaction to stress and help regulate many of our automatic processes such as digestion, the immune systems, mood, emotions, sexuality, energy storage, and expenditure.

Not to get too much into biology, but this may help us understand more about the reality of stress and the domino effect that occurs from the inside out:

"Adrenocorticotropic hormone (ACTH) is transported by the blood to the adrenal cortex of the adrenal gland, where it rapidly stimulates biosynthesis of corticosteroids such as cortisol from cholesterol. Cortisol is a major stress hormone and has effects on many tissues in the body, including the brain. In the brain, cortisol acts on two types of receptor – mineralocorticoid receptors and glucocorticoid receptors, and these are expressed by many different types of neurons. One important target of glucocorticoids is the hypothalamus, which is a major controlling center of the HPA axis."

"The corticotrophin-releasing hormone and vasopressin are secreted by the PVN neurons into the hypophysial portal system stimulate the pituitary cells to produce and secrete adrenocorticotropic hormone (ACTH) into the general circulation. ACTH then stimulates cortisol secretion by the adrenal glands."

Source: Farlex Partner Medical Dictionary

"The combined system of the neuroendocrine units that in a negative feedback network regulates the adrenal gland's hormonal activities."

Source: Mosby's Medical Dictionary

> "A major component of the stress response system, consisting of the hypothalamus, anterior pituitary, cortex and the cortex of the super adrenal gland. The HPA Axis regulates secretion of cortisol from the suprarenal gland in response to stress."
>
> Source: Medical Dictionary for the Health Professions and Nursing

Complicated and intimidating right? This is why we are going to simplify the medical terminology and talk about the adrenals, cortisol, and "chronic stress disease." Who wants to mess up and disrupt the HPA Axis and the hormones?

> *Basic HPA axis summary (corticotrophin-releasing hormone =CRH, adrenocorticotropic hormone = ACTH). The hypothalamus, pituitary gland, and adrenal cortex.*
>
> *The hypothalamic–pituitary–adrenal axis (HPA axis or HTPA axis) is a complex set of direct influences and feedback interactions among three endocrine glands: the hypothalamus, the pituitary gland (a pea-shaped structure located below the hypothalamus), and the adrenal (also called "suprarenal") glands (small, conical organs on top of the kidneys).*
>
> *There are bi-directional communication and feedback between the HPA axis and immune system.* **The HPA axis, in turn, modulates the immune response, with high levels of cortisol resulting in a suppression of immune and inflammatory reactions.** *The relationship between chronic stress and its concomitant activation of the HPA axis, and* **dysfunction of the immune system is unclear**; *studies have found both immunosuppression and hyperactivation of the immune response.*

Studies on people show that the HPA axis is activated in different ways during chronic stress depending on the type of stressor, **the person's response to the stressor** *and other factors. Stressors that are uncontrollable, threaten physical integrity or involve trauma tend to have a high, flat diurnal profile of cortisol release (with lower-than-normal levels of cortisol in the morning and higher-than-normal levels in the evening)* **resulting in a high overall level of daily cortisol release**.

On the other hand, controllable stressors tend to produce higher-than-normal morning cortisol. Stress hormone release tends to decline gradually after a stressor occurs. In post-traumatic stress disorder, there appears to be lower-than-normal cortisol release, and it is thought that a blunted hormonal response to stress may predispose a person to develop PTSD. [20]

Source: http://tinyurl.com/AFSolution

These definitions are a little too medical for the most of all of us... so we simplify the process of HPA Axis dysregulation into stages adrenal dysfunction to exhaustion. We should call the effects of living each day with chronic "busy-ness" which results over time in what I call the "chronic stress disease."

Most people—just like me—first head to their doctor when they feel off and experiencing frequent unusual levels of fatigue. We ask our doctor why we feel so tired all day, why we've gained weight so quickly, what's with the excessive brain fog and sudden onset of depression? Perhaps the traditional medical system isn't the route to take when having these common symptoms as most people leave their doctor's office with a prescription for anti-anxiety, depression, or a sleeping aid.

I wish we would get answers to help us understand why do we have weight gain and fatigue, what is the root cause of all of our internal health problems, and so on? I am not a doctor, but I wanted to share my experience, my background, and my journey with you.

I am now on a mission to help others who may experience similar symptoms and help others get off this dead end road.

A detour is needed.

A revision in life in order to continue down a healthy and happy way of living.

Your Greatest Wealth is Health

8

"Your greatest wealth is health actually rejoice in that and live life have fun and relax and I have seen that the closer you get to perfection it feels so much better we are striving to be a better person but the happiness element and confidence in your element give you the confidence to be content and grateful for present in what you have today and I can say that I can improve my health and there is this confidence that what I am doing today is enough."
- Trish Blackwell, The Confidence Coach

When I started participating in local sprint triathlons and then gradually adding cycling, and running, and long-distance events at age twenty-five, I figured out my new favorite hobby and my calling in life besides being a fitness trainer and coach. Through such physical exertion—and the success I experienced—I discovered a new sense of self-confidence and self-esteem. I became known in certain circles as an "athlete" and with that, I developed a reputation.

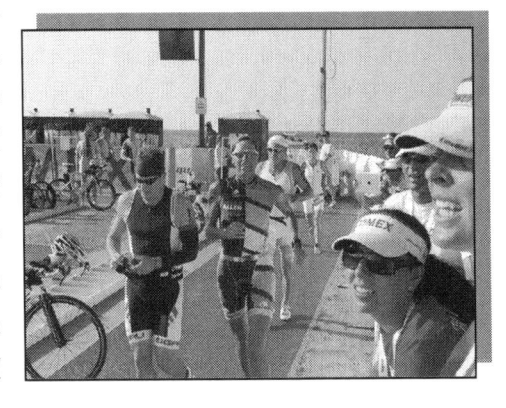

I don't know if my consistent racing commitments were viewed as a positive attribute or a positive reputation to have not. Did people see me as obsessed or was it a compliment to my dedication to training and racing? Both, I am sure.

After few years of doing long distance cycling as the STP and RAMROD in my late twenties, then marathons and doing sprint women's triathlon, I thought I might as well take it to the next level. My triathlon friends from the athletic club where I worked were always training for Ironman Canada each year.

I started to ponder the idea of joining them in 2001. "Why not?"

I was already doing long distance cycling events in one day (200 miles for STP and around 160 miles for RAMROD) as well as marathons (Maui, San Diego, Seattle, and New York City marathons all in 2000). In order to step up to the Ironman distance, I needed to start increasing my swim distance to be in sync with the requirements of the competition. This meant more training time.

In 2001, I completed my first of fifteen Ironman triathlons at age twenty-nine. I quickly got addicted to the endurance training and racing, as well as the thrill of crossing the finish line in such a prestigious and hard-fought event. I become more motivated to train, race, and place in my age group once I started to discover my strength on the bike in addition to my endurance.

In 2003, I joined the Mark Allen Online Elite Triathlon Team, headed by the famous triathlete legend, Mark Allen. I was committed to following each and every workout session on my set triathlon training schedule. The results from my previous years of building up my endurance foundation (all of those long bike rides, long distance cycling events and marathons) by heart rate training (Dr. Maffetone's MAF Training – Max Aerobic Function heart rate ranges), I had built up my stamina engine. My aerobic engine where I could burn high amounts of fat and get faster at a set heart rate (180 – age = MAF). (Read The WHOLESTIC Method manual for more on "MAF" training in the exercise chapter.)

Over the years racing Ironman triathlons, I qualified five times (so far… maybe there will be a comeback in my future once I am healthy from the inside out) for the World Championships every October in Kona, Hawaii. Between 2001 and 2013, I had a few setbacks with accidents as most athletes do over the years which only added to my overall stress, such as bike crashes and surgeries.

As of the writing of this book, my personal journey and my Ironman career may have ended with my participation in the Ironman World Championship in October 2012. I have temporarily retired or rather forced to put my endurance training and racing on hold since I completely exhausted my adrenals. I put myself into such a big hole that I am still healing and recovering from the damage and the aftermath of the internal earthquake I created from not seeing the red flags along the way. I had to hit a roadblock in order to take a different turn onto a new road. Which way will I head now? That is still to be determined. Now, I listen to my mind-body and follow what it tells me to do.

I love the long training workouts as it was time to reflect on life, solve work problems, create ideas, to dream and to totally unplug. My creative brain comes alive when I am on my bike and on long runs. Side note: I usually don't find the zone when I am in Masters Swim workout (adult lap swimming workout with a set workout and send-offs on the board and our coach overseeing our performance.)

When I swim, I am overly focused on every swim stroke and my technique (similar to playing golf- which I say I will never play golf until I stop swimming.) I call swimming "my area of opportunity" rather than a weakness or something I am bad at. It is an area I can improve on and learn more how to excel. Racing can be addictive since we triathletes love to test the limits of our strength, endurance, power, and speed. For me, I was able to do all of that while still staying in my aerobic endurance heart rate ranges where I am efficient at using fat for fuel – not carbohydrates/sugar as we touched upon earlier.

Another type of stress I was putting on myself was the expectation to look a certain way as an athlete and trainer. I was driven and dedicated to looking the part or by my definition of an athlete being lean and strong. Most women tend to obsess about the way their body looks and end up with a negative self-body image. I've always hated my thighs and calves, no matter how fit I was. My thighs seemed too fat and too large from my perspective, plus I always felt I needed to lose an additional five to ten more pounds to be at my "ideal racing weight."

Before my fall out, I would try to lose weight by drinking too much Bullet Proof coffee all morning (coffee with grass-fed butter and coconut oil) and then try intermittent fasting, which is not good if you are already stressing your adrenals. As you should understand by now, you can't add any type of stress to an already stressed body and mind. Extra coffee/stimulants will only add to the turmoil. Fast will be interpreted as another emergency situation to the brain or rather the body's emergency response team – the HPA Axis.

Each year, I continued to race at least one major Ironman triathlon in order to qualify for Kona, participate in local long distance (100 miles or more) cycling events, and running races. After the summer race season ended, I would then transition to the triathlon off-season to only continue with training and racing one or two marathons (26.2 miles) and the North Face 50K trail run (December). My triathlon off season was not months of resting and recovering. True rest was seen as what a lazy person would be doing each day; sitting too much and not moving. Not for me, thanks. I don't like sitting for very long and being still.

Plus, I need to be outside breathing the fresh air. Who needs a real offseason filled with more recovery days? Apparently, I did. No matter how talented an athlete you are, however, strong you have become, or how fit you might be, your body *has* to rest. We are designed to balance our rest and digest nervous system with our fight or flight one.

In 2006, I left a high-end, large, private health club and hotel after working over ten years as an assistant fitness director, top personal trainer, group fitness, and Pilates and yoga instructor. During those years, I developed unique group training and programs such as "Fit Life 6-week weight management program" and "PE 101" plus an outdoor run group.

After a while, my creative and ambitious entrepreneur management personality wanted more. Rather than working for a large health club that the top management didn't respect or appreciate what services I was bringing to the fitness department as well as the relationships and community we were creating, I wanted to create my own all in one studio.

My dream was to offer a fitness studio with personal and group training, spinning, Pilates Reformer, and yoga, plus treatment rooms for Active Release Technique (ART), massage treatment, and acupuncture. As a personal trainer, I wanted to train clients in a stress-free environment without distractions and lots of people (plus people using the fitness equipment incorrectly stressed me out.). I had a vision of "if you build it, they will come." I didn't create the best-detailed business plan. I trusted my gut and went for it. Not the best idea, especially in high-end Bellevue. I assumed my years of being a top trainer and triathlete in the Bellevue-Seattle area would help me be successful, but I also had to run a business, as well as be the head trainer.

After a year of renting space in another training studio and then a year renting a small 1,200 square foot fitness studio to train my own clients privately, I jumped the gun when the opportunity came to move into a larger space three doors over. In 2010, I followed my heart's desire by expanding my studio into a 3,350 square foot fitness studio in the center of downtown Bellevue.

Stressor Alert:
- *Running my own small business and being in charge of all aspects of my own employees: one*
- *Managing trainers to teach group training sessions*
- *Trying to grow, expand and market personal training business to new client base*
- *Renting space in an extremely high-rent district (now up to $7,300 per month, plus overhead, utilities, etc.) that increases every year*
- *Operating a fitness studio in a highly-competitive market*

I'll admit when I first opened my fitness training studio, I definitely was ambitious and focused on becoming the first TRX circuit training private studio. TRX was born in the Navy SEALs as Randy Hedrick created a training device to allow the SEALs to do strength training while at sea. TRX Suspension Training is bodyweight exercise that develops strength, balance, flexibility and core stability simultaneously. The TRX leverages gravity and the user's body weight to complete hundreds of exercises that we implemented into our new group training sessions, but we ended up doing fifty minutes of just TRX based exercises for the first two years my studio was open.

My major business plan error was that I was branding someone else's product and not creating my own. Quickly, everyone was branding my studio, Fitness Forward, as the "TRX workout" studio. TRX Suspension training was a brand new workout tool when I opened up in 2010. I wanted to be unique in creating TRX Circuit Training. I should have started my own Fitness Forward Group Training workout, though. I was trying to be a trendsetter. We jumped on the band wagon early to be the "trendsetters," but as the novelty wore off, our reputation of being the TRX Studio lost some clients. I loved using a variety of workout toys such as kettle bells, sandbags, bodyweight, BOSU, and weights to use for training clients, but now I was stuck with the title of TRX trainer.

The excitement eventually wears off when you're offering the newest and latest trend. The "what is new" eventually ends, then you must evolve and develop another unique product. One must always keep one step ahead of the current trends and fads, especially in fitness.

I now had another stress of reinventing my business model and my fitness studio.

Fitness Forward Studio does deliver fast, effective total-body workouts to build the core, increase strength, boost endurance, improves mobility and stability, but it does so not only by using one workout tool. Fitness Forward Studio offers total body workouts for group training sessions as well as shared thirty-minute personal training sessions.

Who said owning a business was easy? Since my rent and overhead was running me nearly $8,000 per month, I had to generate a lot of revenue in order to pay for my trainers, any repairs, purchases of new supplies or equipment, and then maybe have something left to pay myself and hopefully put money away for my 401k. Good luck. I believed in my talent, product, customer service, and the community we had built up over the years.

A caution to business owners: avoid or limit your dependence on coupons such as Living Social or Groupon, as well as monthly programs like a Class Pass that helps you fill up smaller training sessions. These customers usually are not are long-lasting clients and the excessive amounts of coupon clients in our early days was an incredible amount of stress and test of my patience. Thankfully, I didn't continue doing any more group training specials online, even though it did get us exposure.

Stressor Alert: Running your own small business, with incredibly high rent plus creating your own brand is ideal, but also comes with a lot of obstacles to overcome and responsibilities to be successful- and to survive.

I started work in the early morning until late evening hours. On top of teaching most of the total body group training sessions and personal training, I was also coaching clients for triathlon and running events. More is better right? In order to be successful and make any type of profit, I had to create different sources of revenue, but I was also doing what I loved, so my job wasn't really "work" to me.

On top of my business responsibilities and client schedule, I continued to train for Ironman distance triathlons at a very competitive level, following my weekly training schedule from Mark Allen online. I fit my training sessions in between my work duties, as well as into the weekend. Work, train, eat, work, sleep, and work.

Stressor alert: Running your own small business more than full-time hours plus add another twenty hours or more for training for an Ironman is not always good for your health.

I will always remember the conversation I had with the owner of the hot yoga studio that recently moved in above my studio. The owner asked me to go get manicure/pedicure to talk about our business plans. She asked me the perfect question for a fitness business owner that will forever be repeated in my head until I close my business:

"Are you starting a new business or are you opening a place for you to work?"

What a perfect question to ask. I was stumped by it, thinking through my answer. I wondered why I desperately wanted to have my own brick and mortar fitness studio. Did I want the private, quiet, professional environment to train my own personal training clients or did I do it to have other trainers work for me?

As a fitness studio owner with your name connected to the business, I was also the face and voice of the company. Most days, I was a one-man show if my personal trainers were not available to teach their group session. The business and lease/rental agreement were all on me, as well as our house. After reflecting on my goals, mission, and vision, I decided I wanted trainers who would work with me and also be motivated to create an amazingly supportive community, as well as a top-notch, high-end, boutique fitness studio with Ritz Carlton-esque customer service.

Stressor alert: Being a one man show is not ideal. Delegate. Create a team, a tribe, and a community where everyone has a stake in the business' success.

I would pack my days full with client appointments, computer work, accounting, marketing, and my own triathlon training, plus yoga three to four days a week to "unwind" and "relax." What did I know about really slowing down, letting go and relaxing? Before I knew it, it was bedtime (which was 9:00 p.m. back then) to repeat the schedule the next day.

> "SLOW DOWN and enjoy yourself a little more, don't be
> so serious, life is not a race."
> – Christiane Lemieux

This everyday schedule was "normal" to me. I thought this was how I was designed to operate and to succeed in life.

Stressor alert: We need seven to nine hours of sleep each night. So, when you go to bed at 9:00 p.m. and wake up at 3:45 a.m., that doesn't allow enough time for your body to rest, repair, and recover. Nowadays, I am in bed by 7:30 p.m. some nights. No one messes with my sleep.

I was aware of the importance of sleep and relaxation, but I thought I was getting enough at the time. I was doing yoga two to four times per week and crammed yoga classes into my already packed schedule. I was adding more activities in my day in order to relax, rest my nervous system, and improve my flexibility and mobility. However, the opposite benefits were most likely occurring in my body; two to three yoga classes took four to six hours in my week, as well as cutting into the small amount of quality time with my husband.

Stressor Alert: Yoga is extremely beneficial for your mind and body, but make sure you are not creating extra stress in your life by trying to fit in into your day if it is already too packed and overscheduled. Plus, too much of anything can be toxic. You are better off decreasing your time in another workout or replacing it with yoga, especially if you are anxious, tense and have difficulty unwinding or being still.

As the owner, not only are you managing the day-to-day details, you're also keeping up with online marketing, social media, blogging, website development, creating content, attending networking events, getting new clients, and more. Failure was not an option for me. I may have been overextended, yet I didn't want to give up my fitness studio because I would have felt like I'd failed. The first few years, my peers were secretly watching to see if I would succeed. I had a reputation as one of the top fitness trainers and athletes in the area, but could I succeed as a business owner, as well?

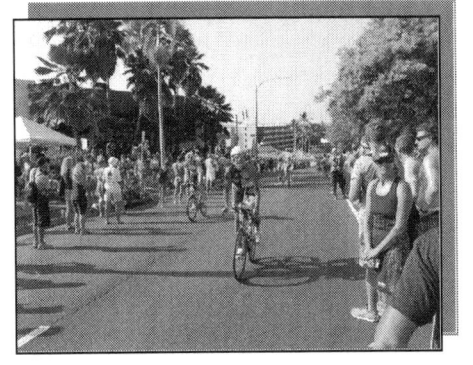

"As long as you are worried about what others think of you, you are owned by them. Only when you require no approval from outside yourself can you own yourself."
- Neale Donald Walsch

Every day, I am driven and motivated to succeed, yet I always struggle to find enough hours in the day to accomplish all of my goals and my list of responsibilities. Back then, my solution to find more time was to cut back on sleep to get more work done at night or first thing in the morning (4:30 a.m.? Really?) The days couldn't start any earlier than they did at the time and I could not fit anything else in my schedule.

On top of my crazy lifestyle, training schedule, and a shortage of sleep, I became overly strict (or perhaps obsessed) with low carb eating by only having one big meal per day. I would have my delicious and favorite way to start my weekday mornings is Bullet Proof coffee (Dave Asprey's fat coffee: *see below*), then have one big meal in the afternoon after my workout session and then back to work for my evening shift.

I can easily do fifteen to eighteen hours of intermittent fasting (IF) almost every day without trying- as the higher fat meals filled me up for hours. Higher healthy fats, moderate amounts of quality protein and lots of vegetables for carbohydrates (and fiber) works best for me – even today, but fasting is not ideal when you are experiencing chronic stress as myself. Adrenal dysfunction and intermittent fasting do not mix.

The fasting could have been the "straw the broke the camel's back" for my fall out in the start of 2013. Be aware. Eat best for your metabolic type and only try intermittent fasting if you are not under excessive stress- as your body will only interpret fasting or not eating for long periods of time as another threat and go into an emergency mode in response to the situation. No more triggers to stress allowed when you already have a huge long list of them.

Stressor Alert: Intermittent fasting is not always beneficial for women and stressed people. Sadly, we often are not aware we are an overly-stressed person until you are forced to the sidelines like me.

In order to stay in a fasted state all morning and to keep

alert after not getting enough sleep, I would overdose on too many cups of my favorite fat (Bullet Proof coffee) for the first half of the day and then eat a big salad for lunch around 2:00 p.m. (after my noon Masters Swim workout or afternoon bike ride) That would keep me full for the rest of the day. The result was fasting for over fifteen hours to help my digestive system rest and body use fat for fuel. Fasting occasionally isn't a bad thing (see Jimmy Moore's new book coming out) but it should not be done every day, especially if you are stressed/busy, female, and have a heavy volume of endurance triathlon training.

Stressor Alert: My fasting experiment was actually adding another type of stress to my already fatigued adrenal glands and hormonal system. Stress comes in different forms: chronic cardio, finances, family, work, nutrition, and more.

At the end of 2012, I felt like I was in the best racing shape of my life. I was metabolically efficient, a fat burner, and had amazing endurance levels. My food plan was (and still is today) low-carb/high-fat primal Paleo type of food plan. Eating healthy fats makes you feel full and satisfied for hours; thus causing you to eat less during the day. Even though I felt strong and fast, I didn't know my body was gradually breaking down from the inside out. I was sluggish on bike rides with dead exhausted leg muscles even when I'd barely put on any mileage.

As a long time athlete who trained by heart rate, I noticed mine was soaring when I was on my bike and run speeds when it typically was ten to thirty beats lower. What had happened to me? I was a hardworking, dedicated triathlete, trainer, coach, and fitness studio owner? This wasn't right. This wasn't how things were supposed to be. I knew my body was off and I needed help.

Stressor Alert: Consuming a high-carb diet with processed foods, gluten, and sugar creates stress in your digestive system and could lead to leaky gut syndrome. A low-carb/high-fat primal Paleo real food eating plan is ideal for balancing blood sugar levels which reduces stress in the body.

I was always learning and growing in my industry... one step ahead of others often since I was often thinking outside of the box and challenging traditional textbook theories. Fortunately, I was doing testing client's metabolic efficiency (ability to burn fat during exercise and at rest) in my Fitness Forward Studio using the "New Leaf Metabolic Cart" starting back in 2005 (sadly, the company got bought out by Lifetime Fitness and we can no longer use the carts.) I started listening to Sean Croxten's "Underground Wellness" podcasts in 2010 about functional medicine, gut health, and real food eating.

In 2012, I followed another educator and blogger, Ben Greenfield then soon joined his twelve-month program to become a certified Superhuman Coach.

My point is, I started my education process of underground health, fitness, and nutrition long before mainstream media spoke about it and before I started to experience all of these health problems first hand. I became my own case study before I had any prediction of what my future had in store for me. Paleo, gluten, gut health, heart rate variability, thyroid health, depression, parasites, adrenals, and metabolic efficiency were all something I was learning about in order to help others. Then, it was my turn to be the client.

My lifestyle habits, mindset, and attitude really needed an adjustment as my "normal" wasn't an acceptable way to operate daily life if I was going to continue living.

"Transformation is often about unlearning than learning

– Richard Rohr

- I don't need to race to and from each life event as if it were a contest and ending each day by crossing the finish line and heading to bed.
- Each day, I should feel successful, confident, and happy on the inside and outside no matter what the situation is that day.
- It is okay to give myself permission to slow down and not feel guilty or anxious if I'm a little behind or off schedule.
- I don't need to speed through my daily scheduled appointments as if they are timed transitions in order to get to the next event as quickly as possible. I've always tried to be efficient and not waste any time between events.
- Life is not a competition. I don't need to approach each day with the pressure to win by completing everything on my list or in training schedule… and then some.

We should face each day as a new beginning on our journey. We need to enjoy the moment; focus and being more present with the people in our lives and deal with normal tasks one at a time.

Slow down.

Breathe.

Look at your surroundings and observe life.

> *"Maybe the journey isn't so much about becoming anything. Maybe it's about unbecoming everything that isn't really you, so you can be who you were meant to be in the first place."*
> *– Summer Saldana*

Every day may unpredictable as the trade winds in Kona—and yes, sometimes experiences in life are out of our control—but how do we react to situations is the lesson to be learned especially if you are easily worked up, tense and stressed as I was in the past The positive takeaway is we can choose how we approach and handle the situations we face daily. We always need to be prepared to deal with various challenges and struggles with the right attitude and a sense of calmness.

Stressor Alert: How we react to situations is a major part of the stress we can accumulate each day. Typically, we become negative, short-tempered, and anxious. Instead, we should take a moment to assess what's going on and breathe before us to respond or react.

We have our own built-in Emergency Response System we can overwork or abuse or take advantage or else they will quit on the job. You understand now how we only have one life and we should see it as a journey. We may need to remind ourselves frequently that we need to own our health from the inside out and it is our choice which road we will travel on our adventure. One technique I talk a lot about in my chapter on stress in The WHOLESTIC Method and on my podcast, *The WHOLE Athlete,* helps you monitor your daily stress levels. With new technology, that is always improving and evolving, we now can measure our resiliency to our own stress in life. We can simply do this by using a Bluetooth (we use MYZONE monitor) heart rate monitor and the "Sweetbeat Life" app on your phone to test what is called your heart rate variability or "HRV" for short.

Remember, my mission for sharing my personal story is only to help you help yourself- and avoid getting to the point I did with my stress response system. I am here to save you from heading into what some people call (Dr. Lam and Dr. Kalish) Stage Two adrenal dysfunction or worse, Stage Three, adrenal dysfunction." You need to get serious about your health and future well-being, because from my observations, we all need to focus on ourselves more often.

Today, start to take control of your own specific stressors by first identifying what sets off your frustration, anger, and anxiety.

What are your triggers?

Make a chart of what moves your soul.

Make another list of what sucks the energy from you.

Next identify your "Energy Robbers" as Dr. Wilson describes in his book "Adrenal Fatigue: The 21st Century Stress Syndrome."

Our "Energy Robbers" could be a person, something at home, our workplace, our environment and even the food we eat.

Make your list or create columns now or use my The WHOLESTIC Method workbook for more in-depth questions to help you develop your roadmap to success in life and sports performance.

Giving Your Body a Tune Up   9

"Anxiety happens when you think you have to figure out everything all at once. Breathe. You're strong. You got this. Take it day by day."
– Karen Salmansohm

We can relate the way we treat our body to how we treat our own cars. As responsible car owners and to keep our car running smoothing on the road, we need to get tune-ups, oil change, replace parts, and even get our car detailed from the inside out occasionally. When we drive our car on the road, we have speed limits with signs, traffic circles and speed bumps to force us to slow down our speed. We see construction on the road that requires us to take revisions and find alternative routes to continue on our journey… and sometimes we hit an unexpected dead end.

Now, how can you take what you learn about how you treat and drive the car you own and use each day (to keep your car running as well as avoid speeding tickets and accidents) and put it toward the positive maintenance of your own health? Why do we treat our cars better than our own body? We must reboot our internal system and *work in* before we start *working out*.

The big question is how can we train for our own personal Ironman race while maintaining our internal health and happiness?

I am going to share my personal story with you on how I had to start working from the inside out to figure out the root cause of my health problems and begin repairing them. First and foremost, I had to start taking responsibility for my body, health, and mind in order to continue on this journey called life. We only have one body and one life, so let's not take it for granted. You can always trade in your old car for a new one, but you can't trade in your body for a replacement model.

We constantly are asking our body to respond to various stressors we come across in our daily lives in different forms such as physical, emotional, financial, environmental, and more types of stress that are all around us. How we respond to the stressors that come at us all day long is something we can learn to control and monitor. Our adrenal glands respond to the stress by secreting the main stress hormone called cortisol resulting in excessive release of cortisol in the body over time. This will lead to a domino effect of internal chaos.

Check out Dr. Terry Wahl's video lesson and her blogs at: http://terrywahls.com/

The adrenals also play another role besides responding to stress as our "Fight or Flight" and releasing the hormone cortisol as well as the hormone DHEA and epinephrine. These hormones also regulate our heart rate (stressor alert – higher heart rate at rest and in exercise sessions), immune system (getting sick more often or more frequent colds?), energy storage (gaining weight for no reason?) and other roles we will discuss in later chapters.

Again, I am only sharing my experience. I am not a physician, functional medicine doctor, or naturopath, but I can refer you to my team of practitioners that helped me get through this stress disease.

There is a connection to our health with our constant chronic daily stress from living each day as its own race by the way our society promotes our busy lifestyle (and always being connected to social media, emails, or text messages). The level of "busy-ness" we thrive on each day is also draining and exhausting our hormones, specifically our stress response hormone system.

If you do a Google search on "Adrenal dysfunction" or "HPA Axis Dysregulation" you will have a huge list of websites, healing programs, blogs, and books to review. Adrenal dysfunction and HPA Axis dysregulation is currently a growing epidemic in our society and also very undetected in most individuals, but I can spot the symptoms in each person I guarantee has low or high cortisol levels as well as a domino effect on the rest of their body systems. This is my motivation and why I am sharing my story. I want to help others avoid the "chronic stress disease" epidemic and evade the disaster my body and mind has experienced.

I asked a few of my mentors for their definition of chronic fatigue issues since different practitioners have various opinions:

> *"Emotional, dietary and inflammatory stress accumulates and in order to combat these issues, our neuroendocrine system responds. Adrenal dysfunction describes the moment that the adrenal gland's ability to respond to all the stress in our lives starts to fail. In a normal individual with healthy adrenal hormone levels, the brain and adrenals link together in what's called the HPA (hypothalamus pituitary adrenal) axis to respond to stress, rest, and then relax, again to respond to stress and relax. When this responding system fails, the brain and adrenals lose their normal system of communication and the person starts to be unable to respond to stress. This is what we call adrenal dysfunction or the technical term is HPA axis dysfunction."*
>
> Dr. Dan Kalish, www.kalishinstitute.com

"There are too many opinions on this [issue of adrenal dysfunction], but some very clear physiologic facts exist. Please help people understand that the so-called "adrenal problems" are all downstream conditions (from the brain). The HPA axis is the key discussion. For more information: http://tinyurl.com/SportsMedicineSpringer.

Dr. Phil Maffetone, https://philmaffetone.com

"This concept has been bantered about for decades. I remember when I was racing as a professional triathlete and feeling extremely fatigued for weeks on end. I obtained all manner of blood tests at great expense and everything was fine. I was a healthy specimen who happened to feel like staying on the couch instead of getting out on my bike. Yes, it seemed like I had adrenal dysfunction. I read all the books about how the stress response worked, including a good one called "Adrenalin and Stress" by Archibald Hart, and also the work of Hans Selye, father of modern stress research. Yes, what a bummer it was to have adrenal dysfunction, like having IT band syndrome. Just recently, Dr. Cate Shanahan delivered a memorable comment to me on this subject. She said, 'There is nothing wrong with your adrenals per se, **it's the stimulus you are delivering to them that is the problem. Overly stressful training, traveling, and lifestyle patterns overtax the adrenals and they start to under produce important hormones.** They are working as nature and genetics intended. If you are getting worn out, your body will find ways to slow down. It's an important perspective to adopt in general, especially when we overuse prescription drugs...to combat lifestyle-related problems.'"

Brad Kearns, Author, Speaker & Podcast host

"Adrenal dysfunction" is a misnomer; a more complete way to encompass the gravity held here is Hypothalamus, Pituitary, Adrenal Dysregulation, or HPA-D. This system has a global effect on most all tissues and cells within the body; therefore, it is unlikely to heal any chronic issue without deep respect and addressing of these systems."

Jator Pierre, C.H.E.K Practitioner www.wehlc.com

"In healthy, low-stress individuals, this entire HPA axis feedback loop works in harmony. But when cortisol and norepinephrine are chronically overproduced, the HPA axis eventually becomes desensitized to the negative feedback telling it to "calm down," leading to chronic stress on the hypothalamus, pituitary gland, and adrenal glands. Eventually, this leads to the neural failure that eventually causes all the nasty adrenal dysfunction issues you learned about called HPA axis dysregulation."

Ben Greenfield, https://bengreenfieldfitness.com

Our brain is the "commander in charge or the "Central Governor" as well-known scientist and educator, Professor Tim Noakes, from Cape Town, South Africa, discusses in his books, blogs, and podcasts. Over time, our stress response system can get broken down from over stimulus and constant overuse. We will dive into what are forms of stress and even more in my The WHOLESTIC Method manual were I discuss in great detail the role of eight elements that impact our ability to burn fat, optimize our health, and improve our performance.

For more information visit: http://www.famousscientists.org/tim-noakes/ or http://www.thenoakesfoundation.org/prof-noakes

Whatever you want to term the root cause of having exhaustion, brain fog, unexplained weight gain, trouble sleeping, gut problems, and hormone imbalance, it is coming from an overload of chronic stress in all forms and living each day as another race. Over time, we have a breakdown in our internal communication system that leads to an imbalance in our internal regulators or manager's system overload. Being a successful individual in life and athletics should not be defined as being an invincible superhero that can do everything top notch and reach peak performance daily. Saying "yes" to everything and everyone is not a sign of success, wealth, or health.

We need to re-define what is healthy and what is worth doing for our well-being in life and sports. Maybe I am not a lazy person if I lay down for twenty minutes or if I skip a workout because I don't feel energized. Perhaps, I am not a bad business owner if I am not always at the studio during prime hours. The art of being busy isn't the key to being successful or healthy.

Our adrenal glands are small—about a size of a walnut— and sits above each kidney (www.hormone.org). The adrenals produce hormones that help the body control/regulate blood sugar, burn protein, and fat, and respond to stressors from a major injury or illness. The most important role of the adrenals is to manage our stress levels daily. However, what if we demand too much on our stress response system and overtax the adrenal glands?

Well, the domino effect begins…

My condition I have been healing from over the last three-plus years is related to the breakdown of how the hypothalamus in the brain interacts with the pituitary and adrenal glands… a negative feedback loop. The dysfunction or also termed the dysregulation, of the Hypothalamus-Pituitary-Adrenal Axis or for short, HPA Axis, as previously described and defined. I am not a biochemist or a medical expert, so I like to simplify the message by saying it is the result of living life each day as its own race.

To oversimplify the concept of HPA Axis dysregulation, the phases are termed in three stages, according to Dr. Daniel Kalish, who created his own model of Functional Medicine and has worked with thousands of patients and trained hundreds of practitioners. The simplified version of HPA dysregulation or the stages of adrenal dysfunction is to test cortisol and DHEA levels to determine level using saliva test or new DUTCH test.

Info from "The Kalish Method" book by Dr. Kalish and http://tinyurl.com/AdrenalTesting

Let's review some theories of the stages of adrenal dysfunction according to both to Dr. Michael Lam (www.drlam.com) who specializes in the research of adrenal issues and Dr. Kalish, as previously mentioned:

- **Stage One**:
  The Alarm Reaction - the body is alarmed by the stressors which lead to an aggressive anti-stress response to overcome the stressors (increase in anti-stress hormones like cortisol). The initial rush of our stress hormone cortisol is high. You are probably under a lot of stress, but more of an enjoyable type of stress as when you are starting college/job or become a new parent. You feel energized and excited, but the secret is to find what I call the "Goldilocks" amount of stress as we need some level of stress. How much depends on your resiliency and

ability to adapt. The right amount of tolerable stress is the volume you are able to absorb and benefit from and then let go or else you transition to...

- **Stage Two:**
  Resistance Response - the adrenals eventually are not able to keep up with the body's demand for cortisol as a result from with living daily with chronic or severe stress. Normal daily functions are executed, but by the end of each day, you feel more fatigued and need to rest more in order to recover. The single organ systems start to be dysfunctional such as metabolic, immunological, and neurological systems. If we stay in high levels of cortisol for too long (Stage One), then we see cortisol levels become lower than normal. Here in Stage Two, cortisol levels drop low and become depleted. If we skip the rest and recover part of responding to stressful situations then we begin to overtax our adrenals. When our adrenals are over-activated too frequently or all the time ("go-go cruise control" lifestyle) the stress hormone cortisol levels will drop—I use the analogy of a leaky faucet. When our cortisol levels are out of balance, we start to see the internal health problems begin such as gaining weight, trouble sleeping, and a low sex drive. (I had it all.) Then, if we are staying in stage two for too long—I was living in it and it became my "normal"—then...

- **Stage Three**:
  Adrenal dysfunction - the adrenals are no longer able to keep up with the consistent and excessive demand for more cortisol production to deal with the non-stop stress,

so they become exhausted. Gradually, the cortisol's output begins to decline. The body goes into survival mode to conserve energy and enters a catabolic stage where we break down muscle tissue for energy. Now, we see chronic fatigue, depression, reduced exercise tolerance, chronic fibromyalgia, and toxic metabolites in the body which lead to brain fog and insomnia. Our single organ systems that were becoming dysfunctional in Stage Two are now becoming even more chronically dysfunctional. This dysfunction begins to spread through multiple organs (the "internal domino effect"). The cortisol levels drop to an extreme low and the body begins to shut down. The stage also involves exhaustion, weight gain, and depression. This extreme exhaustion point is when we ignored all the red flags and signals our body sets off for us to see, but we've failed at recognizing our own distress signals and continued on with our lifestyle habits were actually creating stress. The constantly dripping faucet is now out of control. There is no more water in the well or rather the adrenals are burned out. The adrenals are not really the ones burned out, but the HPA Axis communication system or feedback loop is dysfunctional. Now, we feel tired all day, we're not able to sleep through the night, unable to recover from workouts, and gaining weight.

I personally experienced what Stage Three adrenal dysfunction was all about and I continue to recover from the damage it did to my body. Emotional stress, dietary stress, and inflammatory stressors all contribute to the adrenal hormonal imbalances.

One of the main reasons I am sharing my personal story is to offer "stressor alerts" to help you wake up and gain awareness of your lifestyle habits that may seem "healthy" right now. During the years previous to my final exhaustion breaking point, I had absolutely no clue I was even in Stage One and then eventually adrenal dysfunction.

Sadly, most conventional medical doctors are not trained in these conditions or phases of the adrenal and HPA axis dysfunction so most people leave their doctor's office with a prescription for depression, anti-anxiety, sleeping pills, and/or even hormone replacement, plus they're told to go on a diet and exercise more. Treating the symptoms doesn't get to the root cause, which is: *Why are you having these symptoms in the first place?*

As I've said, we are accustomed to filling up our daily schedules and living a non-stop "on the go" lifestyle without any question. Perhaps, we have become accustomed to being busy or else it is a sign of being lazy or unproductive. We are built to deal with short bouts of stress with our built-in fight or flight emergency response system, but we can't be on overdrive all day long. We get comfortable with the cruise control button on all day. The end result is a breakdown in the "central governor" communication system. The brain isn't able to communicate to the pituitary gland to tell the adrenal glands to react.

In the book, *The Role of Stress and the HPA Axis in Chronic Disease Management*, the author discusses:

> "Research over the past few decades has greatly increased our understanding of the role the HPA axis plays in metabolic and circadian regulation, and how acute and chronic stressors can create discrete patterns of HPA axis dysfunction. *Unfortunately, much of that*

knowledge is either unknown or unleveraged within most health care settings today. Though clinicians trained in integrative and functional medicine paradigms are often more aware of these details, in many cases they are using out-of-date nomenclature or oversimplified explanations that need updating or correcting."

Source: http://tinyurl.com/PointInstitute

"The use of terms like 'adrenal dysfunction,' and 'adrenal dysfunction' to summarize the complex dysfunctions related to the stress response is one such explanation. Though these terms have helped dispel the notion that only extreme issues related to adrenal function (Addison's or Cushing's disease) are of clinical importance, and have become surrogate descriptions for stress-related outcomes, they should now be replaced by more accurate and medically appropriate terms (i.e., HPA axis dysfunction, adrenal insufficiency, hypocortisolism."

Source: "Reassessing the Nomenclature of HPA axis Dysfunction is it Adrenal dysfunction?" by Thomas G. Guilliams, Ph.D.

Let me share my simplified version of what happens to our body systems when we start to experience breakdown:

When we overwork anything, it will eventually get broken or become dysfunctional or dysregulated over time. For example, if we keep using the same swing set day after day for several hours daily; eventually the set will get worn out, the ropes and chains weaker, the seat cracked, and it breaks. If we could find the right amount of time can we use the swing per day without breaking down the set structure, then everything would be all right? I call this the "Goldilocks Effect." Not too much or too little stress. We need a little bit, but not too much... just the right amount. How much is too much stress? The answer for most everything we discuss on my podcast, The WHOLE Athlete, is: "It depends."

We are all unique individuals and no one has the same problems in life. Too much of anything may eventually become toxic, but on the opposite side of the spectrum, too little of anything isn't always ideal either and could lead to deficiencies. Your brain doesn't know the difference between good stress and bad stress. Stress is stress. However, how we react to it makes a difference to our whole health.

We have internal stressors and external stressors... some have "good" effects or "bad" effects. Paul Chek, of the C.H.E.K Institute, talks about what stress does to our body and how we do need some stress to be healthy individuals for life. I strongly recommend reading the book "How to Eat, Move, and Be Healthy" to learn more about how you can improve your whole self from the inside out as he has inspired me to continue learning more natural remedies instead of taking supplements or pills.

The C.H.E.K Institute's tagline is "Implementing the Art and Science of Well-Being." Their principles for improving our health and wellbeing are:

1. "Thoughts: The biology of your body is linked to your mind – healthy thinking produces a healthy body.
2. Movement: Movement is life and life is movement. Exercise pumps your organs, removes waste, improves metabolism, and cultivates energy.

3. Nutrition: Whole, organic foods are eaten according to your Primal Pattern Diet Type fuel your body for success!
4. Breathing: Optimal breathing maximizes THE most important nutrient – oxygen, removes waste, and energizes your body.
5. Hydration: The best solution to pollution is dilution – water is an essential cleaning agent for the body.
6. Sleeping: We don't get stronger when we work out, we get stronger when we rest! 8 hours of sleep each night is essential for rest & repair."

These six C.H.E.K principles are the foundation of their program philosophy and guide all of their educational programs. These principles inspire me as a trainer, coach, and educator to change the way I coach myself, as well as my clients. Learn more at http://chekinstitute.com.

External stressors are any type of stress that comes from around us (outside in) such as sunlight, toxic chemical exposure, or even physical pain from an accident or an injury. Internal stressors obviously come from inside our body, often as a result of our reaction to an external stressor.

An example from Paul Chek would be the external stressors of being exposed to toxic chemicals which then leads to cancer. Then, cancer will continue to stress the body systems even when the toxic chemicals are removed.

Our stressors can come from physical, chemical, electromagnetic, psychic, nutritional, or thermal sources, according to Paul Chek. He is right. Everyone battles these stressors each and every day. Too much or excessive amount of stress, in any form, can throw the body out of balance and lead to multiple dysfunctional body systems. How do we stay in homeostasis or in balance that works for us? It depends on your coping mechanisms.

According to Paul Chek, we all have a risk for a parasite or fungal infection (sounds disgusting). The C.H.E.K Institute has done lots of research on parasites and fungal infections as he believes many of us have an infection that often goes undetected. The most common cause of parasites is *stress*. Go figure. Another fact is parasites feed off of sugar sources/carbohydrates. This is another reason why I must eat a low-carb diet. Once again, that chronic stress and high sugar diet we thrive in each day also can lead you to be an ideal home for parasites. If you have problems absorbing nutrients, this could be one of the reasons. Someone else is sharing your nutrients.

Here are a few signs and symptoms Paul Chek has found to look for:

- Sugar cravings?
- Dry, itchy, or flaky skin?
- Abnormal-looking fingernails or toenails?
- Digestive disorders?
- Chronic fatigue?
- Erratic mood swings, nervousness, or depression?
- Joint pains?
- Brain fog?
- Excessive gas?
- Anal or vaginal itching?
- Sleep disruption and insomnia?
- Bruxism (grinding teeth, especially when sleeping)?

Well, what if you have any of these symptoms of leaky gut:

- ADD and ADHD
- Arthritis, asthma, autism, auto-immune disorders
- Chronic fatigue syndrome
- Eczema
- Failure to thrive
- Food allergies and intolerances
- Inflammatory bowel diseases and irritable bowel syndrome
- Faulty liver function
- Malnutrition
- Multiple chemical sensitivities
- Skin disorders
- Mental health challenges including depression and anxiety

The hard lesson is to learn that being constantly "on," busy, and connected to society is not beneficial for our health and our soul if done in an excessive amount. (At least, that's what I learned from my personal experience.) Actually, I had no clue I was not slowing down and pausing to reset myself or recalibrate my body systems.

I hope you will learn that everyone benefits from stopping the "glorification of being busy" which is a tough habit to break for any type "A" personality—those who don't know how to slow down and be still—such as myself.

Hopefully, after reading to this point, you can take notes and learn from my experience. You can switch out the words "Triathlon" or "Ironman" for anything you are adding into your life that may be enough to spill over into excessive commitment and create a constant state of busy-ness, leading you to live in a constant state of stress. As I've said, too much of anything doesn't always result in a positive experience. Sometimes we reach a dead-end in the road and we need to seek an alternative route.

Which road are you going to take to begin your next journey? It is time to take a detour.

Helpful Links:
Diagnosis and Treatment of HPA Axis Dysfunction
    http://tinyurl.com/DiagnosisHPAA
How to Fix HPA Axis Dysfunction
    http://tinyurl.com/FixHPAA
What is Adrenal dysfunction?
    http://tinyurl.com/AFatigue
Signs of Adrenal dysfunction
    http://tinyurl.com/FatigueSigns
Stress and Insomnia
    http://tinyurl.com/StressTired
Understanding Adrenal Function
    http://tinyurl.com/AdrenalFunction
What Is Pregnenolone Steal?
    http://tinyurl.com/PregnSteal
Intro to HPA Axis
    http://tinyurl.com/IntroHPAA
Salivary Cortisol
    http://tinyurl.com/SalCortisol
Hidden Cortisol
    http://tinyurl.com/HiddenCortisol

To Burn Sugar or to Burn Fat? That is the Question.

10

"You have permission to rest. You are not responsible for fixing everything that is broken. You do not have to try and make everyone happy. For now, take time for you. It's time to replenish."
– Unknown

From my experience as an athlete, I have even more of an understanding about the importance of training the WHOLE athlete or individual to improve fat loss, health, and peak performance. I finally got hit in the head with a knowledge that I needed to make *working in* as important as *working out*.

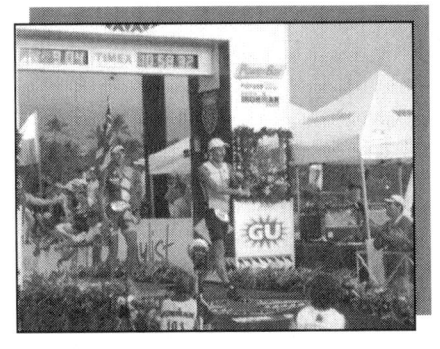

Metabolic efficiency is defined as the degree to which fat is utilized as a fuel source at any given intensity during exercise.

After being in the fitness industry since I was in college, I started to see a pattern with not only myself, but many clients who struggled to lose weight and improve their health even though they exercised consistently. I was not able to help these clients simply by training them one to three times a week. I started to think outside of the box and got curious as to why we are given certain guidelines and rules to lose weight, reduce our risk for heart disease, and stave off diabetes. What we were being told didn't make sense to me as a trainer, coach, or athlete.

How do I burn fat while exercising and training when I am supposed to eat every few hours? Why do I feel hungry after eating what I thought was a healthy breakfast, like having a banana, orange juice, oatmeal, or a bagel with non-fat cream cheese?

The human body relies on a combination of fuels to produce energy at rest and during exercise, but we would be more efficient if we taught our body to burn fat over sugar/glucose for energy. We don't want to breakdown our precious muscle for fuel (glycogenesis).

Think of carbohydrates as kindling to fuel your fire and fat as long slow burning fuel. If we just built a fire with kindling – we would have to continue to keep "feeding" the fire. We would be more efficient and require less tending to the fire if we use a large log or a "Duraflame" long-lasting, slow burn source to keep the fire going for long periods of time. We want to spare our carbohydrates used during exercise and especially at rest, train the body to burn fat for fuel. We can change the percentage of carbohydrates and fat we burn (fuel mixture) by how we eat and train.

I talk about this type of fueling and training in my chapter on "Metabolic Efficiency" in my The WHOLESTIC Method manual. My goal has become to not only reduce your stressors in your life but also teach you how to become a better fat burner with my eight elements of The WHOLESTIC Method approach.

I talk more about the hunger, appetite, and fat storing hormones (leptin, ghrelin, insulin, and glucagon) in the hormones chapter in The WHOLESTIC Method manual. My research into metabolic efficiency (ability to burn fat), hormones, and the impact of sugar addiction on our health has probably been a strong influence on my own personal journey, as well as working with so many personal training/coaching clients over the years. We are all dealing with similar problems and after the same goals: to feel great on the inside and look great on the outside, as well as slow down the aging process.

I know men and women alike can relate to the stressors of growing up. We experience various types of life stress from early ages due to expectations, social pressure, and body image. One of the major challenges teenagers face is to accept who you are and fall in love with yourself.

If you're like me, we are always trying to be someone who we are not as trying to get a smaller frame size and be an impossible size four instead of your natural size eight and not fight it. We could help teenagers today learn how to be happy and satisfied with what we were blessed with instead of trying so hard to be different, shorter, taller, smaller, or leaner.

If we could only have the confidence we gain as to we have more experience in life and learn from our mistakes, hopefully, we would not care about what other people think of us. Ideally, we could simply do our own thing and trust our true friends and family to stick with us throughout our roller coaster ride of a life. We learn something (a gem) from every experience in life and hopefully, we pay attention from those life lessons.

Life is a journey. And, everything happens in life for a reason...

> *"It's a journey. No one is ahead of you or behind you. You are not more "advanced" or less enlightened. You are exactly where you need to be. It's not a contest. It's LIFE. We are ALL teachers and we are ALL students."*
> *– Unknown*

You will know more after reading The WHOLESTIC Method program manual that we all became inefficient fat burners. I survived college eating bagels (the best at Bagelery Bagels in Bellingham), hot-air popcorn (sprayed with water and seasoning salt.), Top Raman, and pasta. No fat on anything and minimal protein. I still have a problem eating animal meat, especially if it looks like it came from an animal recently. When I learned more facts, I ate manufactured soy vegan products in order to get sufficient protein. Yuck.

If you haven't heard yet, processed, factory-made foods, sugar, commercial dairy, and genetically modified foods including grains, soy, peanuts, and corn can wreak havoc on your gut health and digestive system which can lead to inflammation in your body which is another source of internal stress. Do you know too much omega 6 fatty acids cause inflammation in our bodies as compared to omega 3 fatty acids which are anti-inflammatory? Remember inflammation is another form of stress.

A lot of the common "healthy" manufactured foods and the "Standard American Diet" (S.A.D.) are filled with having modified organisms likely to trigger a response that causes the body to become progressively more fatigued. Any threat to the body is another type of stress to the body that causes an activation of the sympathetic nervous system of the fight or flight nervous system. Activating hormone fight or flight response hormone shuts down peristalsis because it inhibits the person ability to digest the foods.

By eating a lot of these common processed foods that are really empty calories (no nutritional value) are full of garbage. Many of which have tons of added sugar to make it taste better. What we eat makes a huge different to our entire health from the inside out, not just our body fat percentage and ability to perform our best in sports. Eat real food to reduce stress in the body. The digestion system will appreciate your kindness and love.

Why are endurance athletes taught to consume 300-500 calories per hour and drink twenty-four ounces of fluid to stay fueled up for their races (and training)? I always fought and debated this guideline. I don't want to use sugar for fuel as I have so much stored body fat available to use for energy, but how do I access the fat stores and metabolize the fatty acids instead of just eating every hour?

When riding longer durations, we needed to figure out how to keep fueled up on the bike each hour. A 300 calorie bar with thirty grams of sugar/carbs and a bottle of Gatorade. My stomach and head would explode if I had that now, but back then this was what we knew best.

When I started endurance events after 1995, the "low-carb and high fat" research, metabolic efficiency, and ancestral health were unknown to me and I didn't understand the role of blood sugar and insulin, like I do today. It wasn't something I learn from nutrition textbooks or in college.

I honestly love endurance training. The endorphin high and the clarity of my mind (alpha brain waves) during long, hilly bike rides and the long runs, especially if I kept my MAF (maximum aerobic function) heart rate to burn fat and avoid fatiguing the body made the long endurance training addicting. Not to mention the thrill and excitement on race day when I was competing in triathlons. How do we fuel, train, and perform our best? The high carbohydrate fueling strategy didn't make sense to me and didn't work either in races (GI problems.)

On that memorable, life-changing Saturday many years ago—the faithful bike ride I mentioned at the beginning of the book—the one that changed everything, I had decided to do an experiment on my fueling strategy. How could I burn fat for fuel and not rely on sugar?

I changed my philosophy on fueling the body for long rides, as well as the drive to seek knowledge on my metabolic efficiency (teach my body to burn fat for fuel), particularly how to stop being on the blood sugar roller coaster as I had been for years.

I'd taught my weekly Saturday morning spin class (indoor cycling group workout) and then drove twenty minutes to meet friends to do a long training bike ride for our first Seattle to Portland Bike event. Since I had needed to lose weight (I was higher body fat and heavier back then) and had excess fat to burn off, I decided not to eat anything after the 7:00 a.m. spin class. I don't remember if I had breakfast before class, but I was probably still into believing a banana, bagel, and orange juice was healthy as it didn't have any fat.

At that time in my life, I didn't know eating low carbohydrates or eating higher healthy fats; just the opposite as fat was the enemy back then. We didn't know about being metabolic efficient or what it meant to be fat adapted. Now, we know sugar is not our only fuel available (read lots more in my manual, The WHOLESTIC Method, as this is the main theme.)

Instead, I ended up experiencing my first "bonking" session as I've discussed. The term bonking is when you hear of a marathoner hitting the wall at mile 18 of a 26.2-mile run or when you have no energy to continue due to lack of fuel. A bonk isn't something you want to experience because it means you've depleted your glycogen stores (liver and muscle) and then experienced sudden fatigue and loss of energy.

Often, the typical solution to avoid "the bonk" is to

supplement with sugar such as gels, bars, and sports drinks which are all filled with carbohydrates. If we just trained our body at heart rates where we are able to burn fat (MAF heart rate training or get tested; more about that in my exercise chapter in the manual), we would reduce the chance of experiencing "the bonk."

We want to spare the muscle and liver glycogen levels by breaking down and utilizing stored fat for fuel. Instead, we are trained to "carbo load" before a long training day or an endurance race to top off our glycogen stores. Some of this is needed, but we only have so much room in our storage areas (muscles and liver) and we tend to reach a capacity of our carb storage early on.

While I rested on the side of the road from my bonk, I had a Cliff Bar (high carbs). The high carbohydrate energy bar gave me the vigor I needed to make it back to our starting point because I was a carb burner (or rather a sugar burner) instead of a fat burning machine. My body had been low on carbs and needed more of them to keep my fuel tank filled up in order to continue cycling.

On this day, I not only had my bonk, but I experienced the body's dependency on carbs for fuel.

> "The need for less often result in a life of more."
> – Brian Gardner

Endurance exercise is a stress on our body, as well as a catabolic exercise. All I ate were carbohydrates. I see people who take gels and sugar drinks to keep fueled even on a long walk as in a half marathon which is 13.1 miles, but we really should be able to burn fat at lower heart rates. We throw ourselves out of fat burning and rely on sugar to keep going which is only adding *more stress* to our body.

How are we to burn fat when we eat so many carbohydrates every day?

That fateful Saturday bike ride happened to be my first experiment on fasting and trying to figure out how to burn fat. I had body fat to use as fuel, but how did I use that fat if I was only eating 250-500 calories per hour on a bike ride? How did I use my body's fat storage for fuel and still have energy? My fasting experiment did not work that day because I was on a high carbohydrate, fat-free eating plan.

Now, I don't need to eat anything when I run for two to three hours (MAF heart rate) or bike up to three hours. We should be burning fat when we're training *and* racing two to fifteen hours as our carbohydrate storing is so much smaller than our fat storage. We can't mostly burn fat while training and racing when we're drinking one to two bottles per hour of high carbohydrate drink mix and/or eating a quick energy gel throughout a race.

Personally, I found out the hard way that my body can't consume that much food or liquids in an Ironman Triathlon. I also learned how to eliminate the excess fluids while I was riding the bike during many Ironman races early on in my triathlon career since I was forcing the recommended bottle of fuel per hour, gels, and bars. My belly was bloated with all of this excess fuel and my body was busy keeping my legs pedaling my bike—not available to help digest food—especially "fake" manufactured foods that are foreign to our bodies. If we are training in our fat burning heart rate ranges to avoid getting fatigued before the finish line in a race, then why do we add so many carbohydrates/sugar into our body every hour to avoid bonking?

Eventually, I started thinking of outside the box ways to improve my training, fueling, and performance levels even before having a metabolic efficiency test and before my favorite Generation UCAN and Bullet Proof Coffee were on the market. My mission was figuring out how to use fat for fuel to keep powered up to perform best for life and sports.

We are taught to keep our metabolism elevated by eating several small meals per day. Instead, we put ourselves on the blood sugar roller coaster—another major stressor on your body and hormones—which is the exact opposite of what you want to do if your goal is to be a fat burning machine or (the more proper term) metabolic efficient athletes.

When I was living and racing—unknowingly—with adrenal dysfunction, I was an efficient fat burner or metabolically efficient athlete. I switched my eating style to a lower carb and high-fat type of primal Paleo plan because that type of eating made me satisfied, satiated, and provided steady energy for hours.

Over time, as I became fat adapted, or able to get off the blood sugar roller coaster that required me to eat every few hours to fuel the fire (kindling versus logs) and the lower carbohydrate high fat eating worked for me, my nutrition and fueling strategies changed drastically as compared to the traditional method for triathletes from high-carb to low-carb and higher fats. The low-carb eating is also best for your adrenals as constant swings in your blood sugar levels puts more stress on your body, most particularly, the hormone insulin (fat storing hormone.)

My nutrition was not the issue for my adrenal dysfunction. That came more from my frenetic work and training schedule that consumed me every day, but made me happy at the same time… or so I thought. My stress was coming from the huge monthly rent I had to pay for my fitness studio, as well as constantly working on marketing strategies and growing my business. Trainers always want to open up their own business without any knowledge that you have to actually do more than train your clients. Financial stress is another major factor for my health debacle. I didn't want to fail as a business owner as I had a reputation of one of the top personal trainers in the area, but was I capable being a successful business owner and top boutique fitness studio? The pressure was coming at me daily, but mostly from my own doing. I wanted to be the best studio in Bellevue, Washington, and have the best trainers in town. I thought it would be an easy goal to achieve based on my background, network, and community. These were all stressor for sure.

I needed to change my mindset, believe in my talent and trust my intuition.

"I am in competition with no one. I have no desire to play the game of being better than anyone. I am simply trying to be better than the person I was yesterday."
– Unknown

How does the Saturday bike ride relate to the story of *Life is not a Race* and my adrenal dysfunction? As I became addicted to endurance events and racing, I continued to learn more about becoming a "Superhuman" athlete and coach.

The Superhuman Coach Network started in 2012 by Ben Greenfield, internationally-recognized fitness and nutrition expert. The program teaches how to:

"Unlock maximum performance for your body and brain, and give you a system for using research-proven foods, supplements and strategies to make you unstoppable – whether your goals are to cross the finish line of an Ironman triathlon, compete in the CrossFit games, or just shed a few pounds. It is the ultimate solution for connecting with someone who you can be 100% confident will allow you to achieve your goals safely, quickly and effectively."

Source: http://superhumancoach.com

The Superhuman Coach Network provides a complete online twelve-month education in advanced topics of performance, recovery, digestion, brain, sleep, hormones, and fitness business and also connects you to a global mastermind of expert coaches for your personal and career growth.

As well as becoming a blogger, speaker, podcaster, and metabolically efficient athlete, I didn't know I was also creating a term based on my journey: The WHOLESTIC Method, its foundation from the experience and knowledge I accumulated over my racing and training years.

The WHOLESTIC Method is designed to improve performance in life and sports from the inside out for athlete of all levels in the hopes of preventing or reversing the daily chronic stress that leads to adrenal dysfunction and more health problems.

Elements of The WHOLESTIC Method   11

"Life is ten percent what happens to you and ninety percent how you react to it."
- Charles R. Swindoll

My transformation began on The WHOLESTIC Method when I started to look at the WHOLE person to improve fat loss, health, and performance from the inside out. I discovered from my own experience that we are not healthy by simply exercising every day.

There is more to being healthy than only exercise, so I have put together eight elements of The WHOLESTIC Method to improve performance in life and sports.

As I started to learn more about adrenal health, heart rate variability, and leaky gut, I began to see the importance of The WHOLESTIC Method in order to be a healthy athlete. Even though I was setting my best times in each consecutive race or competition, I was not really healthy. At the time of my last race season in the fall of 2012, my hormones were plummeting and an internal crash was about to launch. In the spring of 2013, when my weight skyrocketed and I became overly-sensitive to any amount of sugar, I realized being a picture of health isn't about crossing the finish line at an Ironman Triathlon.

An important element of developing the WHOLE person from the inside out is paying special attention to the adrenal glands. Again, the hormone cortisol is released when the body's stress alert button is activated by the adrenal glands. This is the familiar adrenaline rush we get when we are hiking and see a bear in front of us, or, more realistically, when we get stuck in traffic and run the risk of being late for work. We then get that "rush" of cortisol all day long instead of short burst as in our interval training workouts.

I compare this constant activation of the adrenal glands to a leaky faucet. If the bathroom sink tap continues to drip all day long, the water supply will eventually go dry. We can turn the water tap off and on after using it, but the water supply isn't designed to be running all day like that. We have to repair the drippy faucet by finding the source of the leak.

Therein lies the rub. We push and push ourselves to the limit, all the while draining our body of essentials we need.

Why do we do this?

Perhaps we need a guidebook to learn how to live life; an operator's manual we're given at birth. We could start programming kids on how to keep playing, laughing, and smiling as they age. In its place, we start sacrificing our sleep, packing our days full, and pressuring ourselves to succeed by the time we're ten years old or younger. Thanks to our society's over-scheduling and over-achieving goals put on kids over what college to attend, what extra-curricular to participate in, or what advanced classes to take can begin the eventual adrenal burn out starting in the teen years.

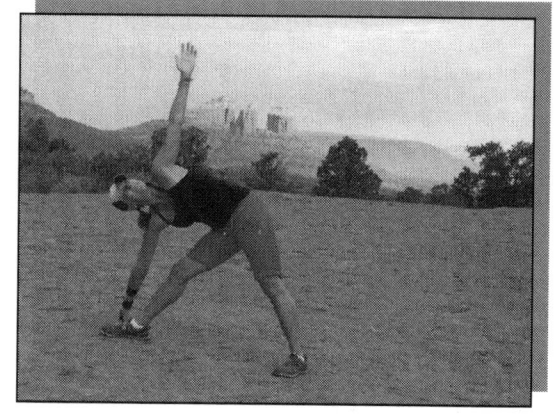

And, from there, life continues on a crazed-spiral through college, career, marriage, kids, and etcetera until we finally slow down when we hit retirement. How is this living life to the fullest? Why do we need to wait until we are over seventy years old to relax?

The WHOLESTIC Method includes eight elements that influence your ability to burn fat, optimize health, and improve performance. In order to increase the WHOLE you for life and sports, we first need to look at various type of stressors that impact all of our eight elements to create the WHOLESTIC you:

Focus on transforming the WHOLE you by improving:

1. Nutrition
2. Exercise
3. Sleep
4. Stress
5. Movement
6. Digestion & Gut Health
7. Hydration
8. Happiness.

Let's briefly review the eight elements that make up The WHOLESTIC Method approach to improving fat loss, health, and performance for life:

NUTRITION:
- What you should eat for your metabolic type
- Protein type, mixed type or carbohydrate type
- Eating real food and organic when possible

EXERCISE:
- Exercise that is best for you based on your health and performance goals
- The "Goldilocks Principle"… not too much, not too little
- Measuring your HRV for recovery

SLEEP:
- Sleep seven to nine hours per night solid sleep.
- Ideally, sleep by 10:00 p.m. until 6:00 a.m., without an alarm if possible.

STRESS:
- Managing your stress levels and becoming aware of triggers
- Measuring your daily heart rate variability with SweetBeat Life app
- Allow "rest and digest" time instead of "running from a lion" all day long.

MOVEMENT:
- To get moving every day (your goal is to complete 10,000 steps per day)
- Do not to sit longer than one hour at a time.

DIGESTION & GUT HEALTH:
- Being aware of your digestion and gut health symptoms as bloated belly, gas, and indigestion
- Order the appropriate lab testing to get to root cause.

HYDRATION:
- Drinking clean water to thirst or recommended half your body weight in ounces of water per day
- Adding a pinch of quality Himalayan sea salt in the morning if feeling dehydrated

HAPPINESS:
- Block off quiet time every day for yourself and enjoy the time alone
- Make time for close friends and family at least once a month

You can dive deeper into each of these eight elements to improve the WHOLE you in my The WHOLESTIC Method program manual.

The Pursuit of Happiness   12

"Your time as a caterpillar has expired and your wings are ready."
- Unknown

I was not raised as a very religious person, but in Hawaii, you cannot help but feel the magical healing powers of the island. I found Madam Pele in my life my first time to the island in 2001 to watch my first Ironman triathlon.

So, who is this Madam Pele who so inspires me?

Madame Pele is the goddess of fire, lightening, wind, volcanoes, and the creator of the Hawaiian Islands. I realized I had to be open to what Madame Pele was telling me when in Hawaii and be respectful of the island god. Instead of being anxious when side winds almost hit me off my bike, I smiled through it and accepted the gift Madame Pele sent to me which was a test or a challenge of my resiliency and reaction. The result of talking to Madame Pele (and singing my magic Kona bike song) was a sense of peace and happiness.

Happiness is one of the key elements of The WHOLESTIC Method manual and program I offer my coaching clients to improve health from the inside out. From my experience, I discovered I needed to learn how to be happy and relaxed and change how I reacted to situations or unpredictable and uncontrollable changes in my intended routine. If a wrench gets thrown into our plan, how can we react in a positive way to it without becoming frustrated or anxious?

For example, I when I had a flat tire before a training bike ride in Kona with my clients. I had a meltdown trying to fix my flat tire with people waiting and watching me. They were fine waiting, but I interpreted the situation differently and threw my tire down on the ground in frustration (trying to rush fixing a flat is not the best way to deal with the situation). The red flag here, by the way, is the inability to cope with stressful situations.

For me to let my mind slow down, I need a week or more in Hawaii. This isn't ideal, obviously, as a vacation is expensive as well as challenging to take time away from work, especially for a business owner. I am learning the importance of finding ways to unwind and unplug in my daily life instead of waiting for my vacation to Hawaii.

How do you decompress, unplug, and re-energize from life…and find happiness again? If you are like me, we often leave a vacation feeling relaxed to only to return to our uptight stressed personalities the few days after a vacation.

We can find ways to be happy at home… I recently started having coffee (love my French press coffee with some heavy cream) outside on the weekend summer mornings. My time in the outdoors, sipping fresh coffee and observing the wildlife play in the surrounding trees in our backyard has become my new secret way to start the day. Sadly, I am not able to make this time during the weekdays and our weather does change in the Pacific Northwest. I know of a new personal sanctuary in my own backyard exists much closer than Kona, Hawaii. We all should have a place near our own home that makes us feel happy… the water, the forest, or the mountains. Find your own sanctuary.

"Happiness is letting go of what you think your life is supposed to look like and celebrating it for everything that is."
– Mandy Hale

We all have different types of chronic stress that hit us every day from unpredictable and uncontrollable situations. Stress comes from not only our running from a lion daily schedule, but also from the food we eat, how we sleep, our digestive health, and more. These varied sources of chronic stress influenced my "Twenty-One Day Sugar Detox" program by eliminating inflammatory foods such as sugar, gluten, soy, peanuts, dairy, and processed foods to morphing into The WHOLESTIC Method.

The eight elements of The WHOLESTIC Method not only help to improve your ability to burn fat, optimize your health, and improve your performance in life and sports, but also to lower stress levels and heal the adrenals. If we reduce our stress levels that come in different forms from external and internal sources, then we may be surprised at how much more energy we have as well as a renewed zest for life.

Most of us do not connect the two together: stress and disease or stress and health. The chronic stress on your body from food, exercise, sleep, toxic relationships, digestion, and other external and internal sources may lead to adrenal dysfunction and eventually adrenal dysfunction if you don't press pause, reset, and find out the root cause of what is doing this to you. Stress is stress and is the root of most of our health (as gut infections) and wellness problems (depression). I didn't feel stressed out or unhealthy, but I suddenly had a long list of food sensitivities and a gut infection.

Maybe you are not doing an intensive Ironman triathlon, but you still have non-stop stress you face each day. Perhaps you can improve the sources (daily schedule) or maybe you can't (boss or co-worker), but let's work on what you can improve or control first. Happiness is essential and one of the important eight elements of The WHOLESTIC Method. If we are unhappy, we probably are stressed and depressed. If we are stressed and/or depressed we may not sleep well, eat well or be motivated to exercise.

The eight elements discussed in detail in The WHOLESTIC Method program are all required to be in homeostasis or balance. Each element depends on the other if one goes haywire, as with our hormones, then a disruption in the rest of the key elements will be impacted, as well.

"Happiness is a choice, not a result. Nothing will make you happy until you choose to be happy. No person will make you happy unless you decide to be happy.
Your happiness will not come to you.
It can only come from you."
- Ralph Marston

Do you have toxic relationships in your workplace, friends, or family life? Perhaps one of your external stressors is coming from the people in your daily life; those Debbie Downers or the people who suck the energy from you. I have had relationships over the years with people that were causing me anxiety and chaos in my life. They were adding another source of stress to my already hectic life. Life is short.

Sometimes we need to clean up our relationships with people who are sources of unnecessary stress. If we could allow ourselves to not feel guilty to terminate a relationship that in the end will make us happier each day… even though the decision at the time is difficult. When you weed out the toxic people in your life, you may find that your stress levels drastically decrease.

Often, you have to be strong and wise enough to let go and move toward new beginnings in life.

We need to be able to start making decisions that may feel selfish at the time but realize that you will be better off in the future. I listen to people each week talk about someone who treated them with disrespect and were speaking without any compassion. My point- remove toxic people from your life if you are feeling stressed every time you are around them – especially if they impact your happiness, self-worth, and self-esteem. You don't deserve that treatment- life is short.

> "Toxic relationships not only make us unhappy; they corrupt our attitude and dispositions in ways that undermine healthier relationships and prevent us from realizing how much better things can be."
> – Michael Josephson

Do you have any relationships that create internal anger, constant bitterness, and new resentment or drain your emotions? Those are all signs that you are dealing with someone that is creating an external source of stress in your life: toxicity. We need to be sure to establish boundaries and make sure they are not destroyed... as my experiences dealing with toxic relationships for my coaching clients. The situation always revealed: "chaos breed where boundaries are absent" (Grace Power Strength blog).

I am genuinely happy when I surround myself with friends who made me smile, laugh, be silly, and feel at ease or rather be myself when I spend time with them. Do you ever notice that some people make you feel on edge and uncomfortable when you are around them...your personality changes? Is steam coming out of your head and your pore? When you clean up your relationships in life you will probably feel a renewed sense of freedom, calmness, serenity, and happiness and act as the true self. You probably don't realize the impact those toxic people are doing to your health or rather sources of your chronic stress. Now, you know how to take a load off of your shoulders.

Start cleaning house with your relationships that may be toxic and impairing your well-being.

Stressor Alert: Make sure you take care of your own happiness and love yourself so you are a better person to be around. We need to love ourselves before we can love others, right?

We need to live with a little yin and a little yang.

Yin and yang? What is that even about? I searched the meaning online as I always say we need to have a little yin and yang, but do I know what I am really talking about?

Let's find out the definition in Chinese philosophy:

> *"Yin and yang: Two halves that together complete wholeness. They are also the starting point for change.*
>
> *When something is whole, by definition, it is unchanging and complete. So, when you split something into two halves—yin and yang—it upsets the equilibrium of wholeness. This starts both halves chasing after each other as they seek a new balance with each other.*
>
> *The word yin comes out to mean "shady side" and yang "sunny side." Yin-yang is the concept of duality forming a whole. We encounter examples of yin and yang every day: night (yin) and day (yang), female (yin) and male (yang), etc. Over thousands of years, quite a bit has been sorted and*

grouped under various Yin-yang classification systems.

The symbol for Yin-yang is called the Taijitu. Most people just call it the Yin-yang symbol in the west. The Taijitu symbol has been found in more than one culture and over the years has come to represent Taoism."

Source: http://tinyurl.com/WhatIsYinYang

Another explanation of Yin-yang, and the symbol is:

The Yin-yang meaning and symbol date back to ancient China and represent the belief that everything in the universe consists of two forces that are opposing but complementary. The Basic Philosophy of Yin-yang:

According to of Yin-yang philosophy, the universe and everything in it is both constant and cyclical. One force dominates and then it is replaced by the opposing force. This activity continues constantly and repeats itself over time.

Examples illustrating the philosophy of Yin-yang includes:

- ✓ *Life and death*
- ✓ *Heaven and earth*
- ✓ *Night and day*
- ✓ *Dark and light*
- ✓ *Health and sickness*
- ✓ *Poverty and wealth*
- ✓ *Cycle of the seasons - cold to hot*
- ✓ *The Yin Yang Symbol*

The symbol of the of Yin-yang, also known as the Tai

Chi or Taiqi symbol, consists of a circle equally divided into black and white sections by a reverse S-like shape. Within the black section is a small circle of white. Within the white section is a small circle of black. Each of the individual aspects of the Yin-yang symbol has a significant meaning, as does the entire of Yin-yang.

Source: http://tinyurl.com/YinYangMeaning

The Chinese principles make so much sense if you let your mind be open to new ways of thinking... just as getting acupuncture and trusting the method. I find this open-mindedness is essential to growth and repair as I find from my acupuncturist, Ying, who helps me repair all aspects of my health, inside and outside injuries.

Now, in traditional western medicine, we look at the balance of our nervous system which is made up of two systems that work together: the central and the peripheral nervous system. The central system is the autonomic nervous system which is divided into the parasympathetic and sympathetic branches. The peripheral nervous system regulates conscious movements.

When we discuss the balance to the nervous system in western medicine we talk about the sympathetic versus the parasympathetic nervous system... our version of yin and yang of western medicine. We talked often about the fight or flight response system which is a result of the sympathetic nervous system branch. The parasympathetic nervous system branch is in charge of rest and digest.

In order to be healthy from the inside out, we need the parasympathetic and sympathetic nervous systems to stay in balance of one another.

Autonomic nervous system: A part of the nervous system that regulates key involuntary functions of the body, including the activity of the heart muscle; the smooth muscles, including the muscles of the intestinal tract; and the glands.

The autonomic nervous system has two divisions: the sympathetic nervous system, which accelerates the heart rate, constricts blood vessels and raises blood pressure, and the parasympathetic nervous system, which slows the heart rate, increases intestinal and gland activity, and relaxes sphincter muscles

The parasympathetic nervous system, together with the sympathetic nervous system, constitutes the autonomic nervous system.

Source: http://tinyurl.com/NervousSystemsInfo

Just another ride on the teeter-totter… the fight or flight response versus the Digestive and Repair Processes. We need to balance breaking down and building up and as we know we can't survive on only breaking down our body systems by living in high-stress mode day after day. If we don't allow more time for our body to rest and repair properly, we are going to pay for neglecting our own health.

I go into the nervous system a lot more in my chapter on Stress in my manual. Most of us are living in fight or flight mode all day as we don't give ourselves permission to unwind and regenerate. I talk about interval training in my chapter on Exercise in my manual, but I am beginning to apply the concept of interval training into our daily lives for myself and coaching clients. Our bodies want to have a moderate amount of stress, fight or flight throughout parts of the day and then hit a speed bump to force ourselves to slow down in order to allow the parasympathetic nervous system to do its job of resting and repairing.

The sympathetic nervous system is also the catabolic-tissue destructive-fight/flight response system. Your lab results (saliva or dry urine tests) will tell you if your cortisol is too elevated, too low, or just right. If the sympathetic nervous system is overworking, you are suppressing the digestion, growth, and repair of hormones monitored by the parasympathetic nervous system. If this system is suppressed constantly, you can't digest foods properly (gut issues and food sensitivities), repair the body (constant nagging injuries), and the tissue-building hormones are not functioning correctly (DHEA, growth hormone, testosterone, estrogen, and progesterone). Why do men get low testosterone? Look at their adrenal health and cortisol levels.

Every day, I see a client or hear about a friend that is dealing with thyroid issues or gut health problems. I hear about so many kids with ADD, ADHD, autism and even depression... why is this growing epidemic in our society at such a young age? The stressors coming from every part of life doesn't have to wait until we are over thirty years of age: physical, chemical, electromagnetic, mental, nutritional, and thermal types of stress are everywhere. The body, or more specifically the HPA Axis starting with their impetration of the stressors by your brain, puts all the good and bad stressors into one funnel then activates the autonomic nervous system and releases the hormones into the body.

The sympathetic nervous system activates our catabolic hormones (breakdown) and the release of the stress hormone cortisol if there is an excessive amount of stress. This is where we find the fatigue, breakdown, depressed immune function, and decreased the ability to repair our body from the inside.

Now, review the other side of the teeter-totter: the parasympathetic nervous system. It releases the anabolic hormones to help digestions, repair, and growth.

How do we find that optimal amount of stress or homeostasis of our nervous system to keep the sympathetic and parasympathetic levels in balance? Everyone is different, so how much stress we can tolerate depends on them. However, we need to take a little and give a little, not too much and too little of anything.

Instead, we keep stressing the fight or flight sympathetic nervous systems (SNS) all day so much more than the parasympathetic nervous system (PNS). We become so overstimulated daily that we end up shutting down the PNS and creating this "out of order" status for our digestion and repair systems. Our hormones become out of balance causing us to be wired at night from not slowing down in the evenings. We can't benefit from the "rest and repair" process that occurs while we are sleeping between 10:00 p.m. and 6:00 a.m.

Ideally, we react to a stressor, activate the sympathetic nervous system, then rest and recover by activating the parasympathetic nervous system. We should be able to be relaxed enough during the day in order to digest the food we eat, eliminate waste, strengthen our immune system, and repair our bodies from exercise. Conversely, we rush around living life as a race, drinking coffee, multitasking, quickly eating processed foods, sitting too much, and drinking too much alcohol. Then, we're surprised when we can't sleep at night.

This snowball effect is common in almost every client I work with at my studio and listeners to my podcast. We all experience some type of stress every day, but how we tolerate it varies to each of us. If we could start by understanding our response to stress, identify our triggers, and then make a plan to address those issues, perhaps we could avoid adrenal dysfunction, low thyroid, gut health issues, or other health problems relating to excessive stress.

We all know the words to the Beatles song "All You Need is Love." In my Paul Chek, C.H.E.K Institute, Holistic Lifestyle Coach program, we talked about what is the "one love" you are willing to experience now. What are you willing to change and grow for today? Do you have a dream of crossing an Ironman triathlon or maybe running a successful small business? Perhaps your goal is to raise your kids to be well-mannered and successful in their own lives.

Whatever your dream may be, to make it a reality, we need to learn how to explore our deeper parts of self. We have to get below the surface and recognize our thoughts, behaviors, and judgments. I am sure you are similar to me and never stopped to think why we do the things that we do. We take the path of least resistance. We do what we think we need to do each day in order to be productive or successful, but we take the shortest road possible in order to not look ourselves in the mirror.

I have spent thousands of dollars on lab tests and consultations since the start of my health debacle in 2013. One of the many things I love about the C.H.E.K Institute and its founder, Paul Chek, is they don't lab tests to know if someone is out of balance. Their practitioners can determine any type of "Yang dominance" indicated in the body as it is characterized by inflammation, redness, swelling, and pain. These are only symptoms of the greater "dis-ease" process the person is undergoing as indicated by self-reporting and their assessments.

At this point, we can connect yin to be anabolic (build-up) and yang to be catabolic (breakdown) when referring to forces leading to unique balance for each individual.

> *"Catabolic reactions usually **release energy** that is used to drive chemical reactions as compared to the opposite where anabolism refers to chemical reactions in which simpler substances are combined to form more complex molecules. Anabolic reactions usually **require energy**. Anabolic reactions build new molecules and/or **store energy**."*

Source: http://tinyurl.com/CatabolicReactions

Let's apply catabolic exercise to anabolic exercise as my exercise schedule each week was based on triathlon training. When I am training for an Ironman, my schedule includes four swims, four bikes, four runs per week plus two strength training sessions per week and sometimes yoga (in the past.)

Endurance exercise is catabolic:

> *"Reaching a catabolic state involves hormones such as cortisol, norepinephrine, and adrenaline. These are useful in burning fat and calories. Many catabolic exercises involve cardiovascular techniques, usually lasting at least twenty to forty-five minutes. Examples are: biking, running, swimming, and playing sports. You will notice a loss of total body mass because more catabolic hormones are released compared to anabolic hormones, which build muscle and mass."*

Source: http://tinyurl.com/AnabolicVsCatabolic

Strength training exercise is anabolic:

"To reach an anabolic state, focus on strength training, which [helps] increase muscle mass. Some of the associated hormones that lead to muscle growth include testosterone... The effect actually takes place when you sleep or rest after workouts. During strength training, you perform exercises that offer resistance using weights and machines. These exercises break down muscle tissue. When you sleep or rest, new and more muscle fibers develop to replace the broken ones."

Source: www.livestrong.com

As we learned from my experience, one of my stressors was a probable result of not balancing the amount of cardio (catabolic) exercise to strength (anabolic) exercise sessions-creating another type of deficit. Not only does Ironman training require you to do long hours swimming, biking and running per week, but it also limits your time available for strength training which I feel is essential for improving performance as well as decreasing risk for injuries and lowering body fat (plus increasing metabolism post workout). Anything in repetition or overuse is not conducive to the health of the WHOLE you. Not only does your body get broken, but your mind altars, as well, from the boredom of being on the hamster wheel.

In The WHOLESTIC Method program, I teach clients to focus on implementing more strength training workouts into their weekly session with higher heart rate intervals when appropriate (depending on their current stress levels). High-intensity interval training involves both the catabolic and anabolic type of exercises – endurance and strength as we do at Fitness Forward Studio. I always tell clients, "You don't need to train for a marathon or a triathlon to shed body fat."

Other elements in The WHOLESTIC Method help you become a fat burner, including the anabolic benefits from strength training. By performing both anabolic and catabolic type of exercise (strength and cardio/aerobic training), it will not only prevent boredom, but also muscle confusion. I always believe if you mix up your type of training, you will confuse the body in order to avoid plateaus and boredom, but also to work on the different energy systems and muscle fibers.

If we continuously shock our body various ways in workout training sessions, we can continue to shed fat and burn more calories after the workout session. Read more about this in my Exercise chapter in The WHOLESTIC Method manual.

Your workouts will also be more intense if you use both approaches alternatively or simultaneously. According to the American College of Sports Medicine, high-intensity interval training (HIIT) involves catabolic and anabolic exercises that boost your endurance and aerobic performance. Doing more "HIIT" training may be more beneficial for some people over sitting on the stationary bike or elliptical for thirty minutes. If you are already stressed out, then we would focus on walking in the outdoors, yoga stretch type of sessions, Barre training (yoga/ballet/Pilates blend), and Pilates.

I asked Vidya McNeil, the business manager for Paul Chek, about the C.H.E.K Philosophy:

> *"What about our lack of rest? That is the biggest issue with most of the people we see in our coaching practice. It just isn't outside ourselves with poor nutrition or electromagnetic solution, it's often what we think and believe, i.e. work hard(er), no pain, no gain. Earliest or inexperienced health and wellness*

coaches tend to fixate on symptoms and then want to "add" too much to a person's regimen in the form of more supplementation, more doing activities, etc. We must help our clients simplify. We raise awareness and we coach to implement strategic changes that are going to help people get the most rebalancing by chunking down starting with what they can and want to do. We coach the whole person who has a challenge, not fix the challenge. The body never lies, even if the mind will rationalize experience."

Source: Vidya McNeill, www.chekinstitute

I try to multi-task too often to get more done at once, but that skill isn't always productive and often lacks focus on each task I am trying to do. I also find the more I try to do at once, the less quality the end result is going to be when I am complete. An example is when I am cooking. My husband is the chef in the family, but sometimes I try to be nice and cook for him. I always mess up our meal if it requires using the stove because I get distracted by doing other chores at the same time or working on something at the same time as cooking dinner on the stovetop. In order to finish a task successfully, I need to focus on only doing that one thing, not multi-tasking.

As I write this book—and in order to focus and get into my zone—I had to turn off my emails and my phone notifications (which are always off now). As I say… "What the F… FOCUS."

Paul Chek teaches an entire section in our Holistic Lifestyle Coaching program on how to find your "1 love" in life. What is your "1 Love?" It is the "why" we do anything? Is it what motivates clients? Is it their Dream as to what they want to achieve or resolve?

First, we have to find a motive to create change; the dream you have of who you want to become needs to be worth experiencing and motivating enough for you to want to create change from the inside out. We don't need to produce more stress by dreaming of becoming something we can't realistically achieve by trying old habits or strategies that didn't work in the past. If you want to stay the same, then keep doing what you are doing now, right? Not only to be want to be around people who bring the best out of us, but also those who do not put the stress on you.

None of us are the same person we were a year ago, a month ago, or even a week ago. I am always growing, improving, and transforming as my daily life experiences don't stop. Those daily life experiences happen for a reason, so find happiness, love, and laughter. The biggest challenge for most of us is to give ourselves the permission to identify and reduce the stress triggers. I want all of us to create a life that not only looks good on the outside, but feels just as good on the inside.

> *"Life can be very noisy. If we allow it, we can live stressed out uptight, in a hurry and on edge. We've got to learn to not let the busyness; the frustration and the stress get on the inside. It may be very hectic on the outside, but deep down there needs to be calmness, a rest."*
> *– Joel Osteen*

A Rehab Center for Busy-ness Addiction?

13

"There is no prize for being the busiest."
- Sobremesa Stories

The healing program that helped me recover the most from adrenal dysfunction, as I've said, was The Kalish Method created by Dr. Dan Kalish. His program integrates scientific lab testing with natural health solutions for fat loss, fatigue, depression, digestive problems, and hormonal imbalances.

A dysfunctional hormonal system seems to be the missing link for most treatment plans in traditional medicine. Based on my experience with conventional medicine, the treatment plan was always a prescription drug. This is what happens when we get metabolically broken and hormonal damaged from our accepted and expected lifestyle habits.

As I've said, The WHOLESTIC Method includes the eight elements to improve the whole person from the inside out based on my experience since we can't repair our hormone imbalance or our adrenals by taking supplements alone. Lifestyle changes, people. We have a choice to make. Taking pills from your doctor or popping healing supplements are not the only solution.

The symptoms from disrupted hormonal, digestive, and liver detox pathway systems lead us to believe they are all "a part of the aging process." We get used to living with our health problems: feeling fat, tired, and depressed for years until such feelings become the norm to us.

We can assume most endurance athletes are typically committed and dedicated personalities. Competitive Ironman triathletes, such as me, often follow our training schedule exactly and never skip a planned workout session even if we feel tired and are experiencing a sluggish day with tired legs. We don't want to get behind on the sessions, so we continue our training program even if our body tells us (loudly) to rest and recover. I would do my slog workouts just to make sure I could enter in the session as complete. I never wanted to show an incomplete session as that would be a sign of failure or laziness.

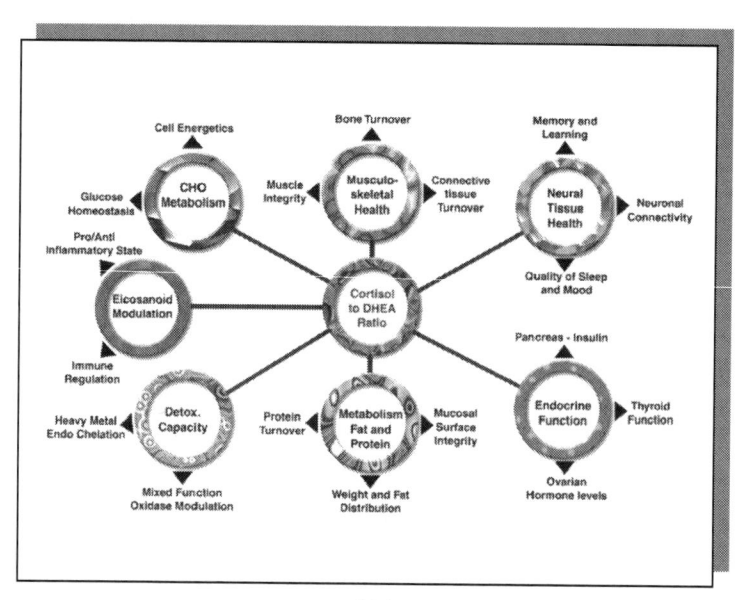

In order to prepare for an Ironman distance race, we feel the need to put the long hours in the pool, on our bikes, and on the road pavement running. The philosophy is often the mentality that if we work harder and are disciplined, the results will pay off on race day. We all want to be even faster, stronger, and more competitive, but at what cost? We think we are being healthy, but in the big picture, we are breaking down our bodies from the inside out. When we are training long hours each week by swimming, biking, and running, we raise our hormone cortisol levels and break down our muscles (catabolic exercise) from the endurance training. Remember, catabolic exercise is breaking down; anabolic exercise is building up. We should have a continuous energy balancing act at a cellular level between the anabolic and catabolic chemical reactions in our bodies just as with yin and yang. Endurance athletes are on a fine line. As I've said before, too much of anything can be toxic and too little of anything could lead to deficiency.

Over time, we may begin to get signs of inflammation in our body, but we continue on because we are invincible. (Or, at least we believe ourselves to be that way.) We may gain weight even though we are training hard and putting in all of the miles, but something doesn't make sense because our workouts take longer to recover from and our race performances start to decline. Stop and listen to your body. It is telling you to slow down, rest, and repair.

As athletes, we discover the internal imbalance and disruption as a bloated belly, difficulty sleeping, a poor recovery, tired dead legs with a high heart rate and excess fat growing on the body that stops us in our tracks. The estrogen, testosterone, progesterone, and pregnenolone levels drop to record lows and are all out of whack, which creates chaos in the internal systems, including your thyroid and liver detox pathways. All the sex hormone levels drop, which you may see in your lack of sex drive.

There is a way to make your workouts and training program not stress the hormonal system. Chronic cardiovascular (long endurance training such as swimming, biking, and running) is a catabolic exercise (breaks down the muscles) as opposed to anabolic exercise (strength training.) Anabolic exercise builds up the hormonal system including increasing growth hormone and testosterone levels, so we all need to incorporate more strength training weekly. Most people, not only triathletes, choose cardio exercise over strength training when they have a choice.

Triathletes can actually improve performance levels by making time for a strength training session over another endurance one. Also, if you are trying to transform your body, a ten to thirty-minute strength training session with cardio blast intervals is going to be more effective than thirty minutes on the stationary bike or the elliptical. Try an experiment: trade out one cardio session for one total body strength training workout with twenty to thirty-second cardio blasts in between sets. Now, watch your fat loss, health, and performance improve. Triathletes will be surprised at the performance gains in swimming, biking, or run training sessions. (Check out my Instagram and Pinterest pages for ideas. Links listed at end of the book.)

Now, you should be more aware of the different forms of stress and how it impacts our total health. You can read more about stress in my companion manual, The WHOLESTIC Method.

The World of Podcasting   14

"Read something positive every night and listen to something helpful every morning."
- Tom Hopkins

Everything happens for a reason in life right? In 2012, I was asked to co-host a new podcast about metabolic efficiency, endurance training, improving performance with low-carb eating and using fat for fuel called, "Fit Fat Fast." The other host was Jon Smith who is passionate about the myths mainstream media teaches us about nutrition, training, and racing for fat loss, optimal health, and performance in endurance sports. We both have backgrounds of eating high carbs and non-fat because it was what we were taught; that fat was bad for us.

Jon originally started his own podcast called, "The Garden Variety" podcast and I was a guest on the show a few times to discuss core, barefoot, and Ironman training. As we both were headed toward learning more about metabolic efficiency for athletes (using fat for fuel and breaking the sugar addiction), we started "Fit Fat Fast" together– until his full-time job took over and I was left on my own.

On our weekly podcast, "Fit Fat Fast," Jon and I talked often about our triathlon race reports, training, fuel plans, and accomplishments, but the most important (and popular with listeners) was our discussions on metabolic efficiency, breaking sugar addictions, ketosis, and eating more fat each day. We both loved the topic of Ironman training, fueling, and performing as a low-carb athlete, but then my experience changed my mission on the podcast, as well as to everyone.

Over time, as my multiple health problems increased, and as my racing and performance decreased, I felt compelled to share my personal story, frustrations, and challenges relating to my performance and fatigue. My institution told me that other listeners could relate to my symptoms and were also seeking guidance to feel, look and perform better.

Suddenly, I was on a personal mission to share my story to the public via our podcast. Did I want to only share my health problems to help others or because I wasn't able to race that year, canceled all of my race plans, but also looked fat, out of shape, and acted depressed? Maybe I overdosed every listener talking about myself. That certainly wasn't the mission of the podcast.

I was obsessed about explaining why I looked and felt the way I did to everyone at my fitness studio, on social media, and on my podcast. Quickly, I was riding high upon my adrenal dysfunction/exhaustion soapbox to anyone who would listen. I knew I wasn't the only one with these unexplained symptoms. I was compelled to explain to everyone I ran into why I was suddenly thirty pounds heavier and not able to train or race. No one cared or really noticed until I said something. I was self-consciousness.

People didn't notice my weight gain as much as I did, but I continued to overly explain the unknown adrenal issue since most people had never heard of HPA Axis dysfunction, adrenal dysfunction, adrenal dysfunction, or adrenal dysfunction, and especially not Pregnenolone Steal. If you want to get me on my soapbox, don't ever tell me to simply take some prescription drugs for depression or anxiety issues to solve my long list of health problems. That was never the solution.

What did I discover by sharing my story?

The response was immediate and comforting. I started getting messages online from our podcast listeners and my Facebook followers. So many people could relate to my struggles and symptoms as they were also searching for answers. Many other folks had trouble sleeping through the night and couldn't understand why they were gaining fat when they were eating real food and training weekly.

Everyone wants to be reassured that the mental, physical, and emotional fatigue they, too, were experiencing was only temporary. Some of my friends didn't understand or believe in naturopathic, holistic, or functional medicine specialists. They were the ones speculating of my condition and treatment. Others thought I needed a medical professional instead of these people who "weren't really medical doctors." The answer was always to take a pill or go get an ultrasound on your liver or gallbladder. I have learned that traditional medicine doesn't always look at the root cause of an illness or even conduct the same lab tests as functional medicine. They don't look at the big picture and/or the WHOLE person. Instead, we are all conditioned to take a pill to stop any and all problems. Medication works sometimes, but often it is a Band-Aid covering up the real problem and cause.

Many of our podcast listeners and personal training clients could relate to my story. I wasn't the only person feeling tired but wired all day, wide awake at 2:00 a.m., muscle fatigue during workouts, depressed, experiencing rapid weight gain, bloated belly and getting a skin rash.

Through offering up a podcast, I was able to reach out to people in need, not just the ones who entered my own fitness center, but anyone from anywhere who listened in downloaded the archive or clicked the link to our show. By interviewing professionals and experts in the field of treating adrenal dysfunction, countless unknown strangers found out they weren't alone and there were other options for them in their own path to healing.

Finding help locally is a challenge, especially if you want a functional doctor or naturopath who specializes in treating "HPA Axis dysfunction" or adrenal dysfunction for endurance athletes- or any level of athlete. I suggest to get started in your quest for knowledge, support, and guidance by doing a Google search in your area or go straight to the top experts I've already recommend: Dr. Dan Kalish or Christopher Kelly at Nourish-Balance-Thrive or even a C.H.E.K practitioner.

You can learn more for free from my weekly podcast called The WHOLE Athlete on my website via www.thewholeathletepodcast.com or search for me on iTunes or Stitcher Radio. I have guest co-hosts on each week to discuss the elements of The WHOLESTIC Method, as well as to break many myths the mainstream media teach us.

I am passionate about sharing my podcasts episodes and blogs to help clear up the confusion on the health information we hear from mainstream media and even some of our medical professionals. Make sure you find a functional doctor to run the proper lab tests to find out more about your metabolic health, cardiovascular health, and more than traditional labs do not cover.

I would have adrenal dysfunction again if I continued listening to clients who were told to eat carbohydrates with a protein to balance their blood sugar when diagnosed with Type 2 diabetes or the food plan for someone with heart disease.

Most of us who do podcasts do it for free because of the passion we have for the subject matter, not because we are funded by any major food or drug company.

As a listener and someone looking for your own answers to your health challenges, you need to keep an open mind and remember to do some digging around for alternative solutions that work for you. It's my hope and goal that my podcast offers that.

A Reflection on my Healing Journey

15

"Obstacles are those frightful things you see when you take your eyes off the goal."
- Henry Ford

Based on my emotional experience and observations with how we treat symptoms in our society, I wrote a blog entitled: *Find the Root Cause and Not Just Treat the Symptoms* - www.fitnessforwardstudio.com/blog. I wrote it during the beginning stages of my exhaustion, weight gain, and depression. These blogs were much more emotional and passionate than I could write today.

We have been trained to go to the doctor when we have a stomach bug, headache, IBS, skin rash, and more. We leave the doctor's office with a feeling of satisfaction. We are going to make some progress and start healing. Then, we begin taking a new medication or following the specific treatment plan from the medication prescribed to us to treat our symptoms. The problem may go away, but often it returns in some form since we didn't actually treat the root cause.

Why do we have this complaint? Where does it start from or what is the cause?

Don't you want to investigate and get to the root cause to determine why you keep getting headaches, bloated belly, or a skin rash on your arms?

Traditional medicine helps treat our symptoms, but I feel we should try to combine non-traditional treatment methods to our healing program. I suggest finding a practitioner who is going to help us investigate our list of symptoms, then dig deeper to research for the root cause. Most functional medicine doctor or a naturopath can help provide a different viewpoint on where the symptoms are coming from as they help find the root cause by asking in-depth questions and request specific lab work.

Instead of renewing your prescribed medication from your dermatologist for skin problems or going to another doctor for stomach aches or headaches, try a different approach that may provide lasting results. Occasionally, we need to think outside of the box and take our health into our own hands and own it.

Perhaps you get a consultation with a nutritional therapist, functional medicine specialist, or a naturopath who specializes in your symptoms. We want to the appropriate guidance to determine the root cause of our ailments instead of getting a simple temporary fix. You may be surprised to discover your symptoms disappear when you heal the gut wall lining, eliminate foods you may be sensitive to, or manage your stress levels. I have learned we need to treat the WHOLE person from the inside out to improve performance in life and sports.

When I was at the beginning of my HPA Axis dysfunction that is generalized as adrenal dysfunction and feeling completely like a huge, beached whale, I was definitely obsessed with researching how to fix myself. Every day, I was over learning and over trying instead of merely pushing the pause button and mellowing out.

How does one slow down and relax when you only know how to race each day to feel successful? If you are like me, a Type A over-achiever personality, I only felt successful when I didn't take a break or slow down during the day.

What does a successful day mean to you?

I needed to learn how to let go of some things in life—like my schedule and accommodating everyone every day—and instead take the time to slow down between appointments and my workouts. Resting on the sofa? No way. I had to give myself permission to chill out and push the pause button more often in order to heal my body from the inside out.

A few years ago, I was introduced to a new friend, Ronda Gates, and her team at Sweetbeat Life - beat healthy. Ronda and the Sweetbeat Life application really helped me understand more about the benefits of measuring and monitoring our daily heart rate variability. We can use the Sweetbeat Life app to measure and monitor our daily stress levels in three to five minutes, our recovery from training sessions to find out if we have been overtraining (and need more rest), and how to monitor our stress/reactions to situations in daily activities like heading to an appointment, sitting in traffic, or even working on my computer over multi-tasking. How can we learn to be still, patient, and calm and focus on doing one thing?

Most endurance junkies and Ironman Triathletes love training and racing and are guilty of overtraining. How often do you listen to your body instead of your training schedule and take a rest day when your body is saying to go for a walk instead of a run? Our body gives us plenty of signals when we need to reschedule a workout, cut the duration or intensity, or even replace it with a rest day. As typical competitive athletes, we usually ignore the red flags and continue on with over training. However, if we would measure our daily Heart Rate Variability (HRV) with the Sweetbeat app to determine if your body needs rest, then we become more aware of the red flags and signals on when to slow down. I definitely had to start testing my HRV daily to determine my progress with healing my adrenals as I wasn't so tempted to increase the duration of my forty minute workouts in the beginning of my treatment. Once again, I share a lot more about how and why to test your heart rate variability in my chapter on exercise and stress in The WHOLESTIC Method manual and the workbook.

In order to improve my metabolism, increase fat loss, optimize my health, and bring back my ability to perform in triathlons, I had to learn how to listen to the signals my body was telling me each day. I need to always listen to those signals and respect them, especially when to take a rest day or have an active recovery workout instead doing a junk slog workout just because it was on my training schedule. I had to ask myself how motivated was I to heal my body, mind and adrenals (as well as gut infection, digestion, thyroid, and hormones) in order to return to racing again, feeling like myself again, and, most importantly, to feel happy.

When the HPA Axis is dysregulated, the adrenals are exhausted as well and the rest of the hormonal and body systems are broken so the healing process isn't quick. I am still healing from my lack of respect for my body and mind for the past four years as I write this or now longer. If I stopped every exercise session, constant activity, and cut my workload in half, the recovery may have been faster, but I continued to push the limits and test if I was ready to begin training again. Honestly, I think I dug myself so far into a hole that by the time I really found out I had health issues. I was too damaged to repair in the typical six to twelve months.

Finally, I am more aware of the importance of different types of performance gains by listening to my body each day. As of today, I am writing this book after my Saturday long masters swim workout before my typical longer bike ride. The old me would have been so stressed to be on time. Now, I take my time leaving swim workout and I don't meet a group to ride as I found committing to meeting other friends to ride at a set time was an added stress to me. I am more self-aware that I don't like to be late to meet people nor do I like to be left behind or fall off the pace of a group bike ride or run.

The new me now rides solo or with my husband on the weekends. The result is a more peaceful workout session for me as the bike or run time is an opportunity to get into my own mind and zone while riding at my pace that feels good for that day (heart rate zones). I know how to listen and respect my body, mind, and health.

A junk workout is very unproductive and ineffective, especially if you are forcing working sessions when you are feeling tight, heavy, sluggish, and tired muscles which actually result in inefficient movement patterns and poor sloppy mechanics. Clearly, some days are more productive if we take a nap, go to yoga, use NormaTech Recovery boots ("Norm" in our household) or take the time to do some mobility work as with the foam roller. I continue to repeat myself (maybe for my own benefit), but we need to listen and honor ourselves by pushing the pause button for one day. Your next workout will be much more effective, faster, and stronger after an active recovery day. If you want to improve your performance levels, then test your HRV daily and stop being tied to your training peaks or training schedule. We all benefit from learning how to be more patient, flexible, and mellow.

Back in the beginning of my adrenal dysfunction, body systems and internal hormonal crash...I was on a mission to explain to everyone the role of the adrenal glands and types of chronic stress as the word "adrenals" was unknown to most people.

Here is that blog post:

On the Road to Healing My Adrenals

Our bodies can only tolerate so much stress (constant activation of the "fight or flight" system) for so long before the stress management team says no more. When the stress management system (adrenal glands) reaches exhaustion from trying to keep up with the constant demands, then something is going to break. Anything we do or use too much of or too little is not a happy ending. I call this the Goldilocks principle.

No longer can the stress hormone cortisol keep up with the output ("fight-or-flight" - sympathetic system) or keep up with the constant stress (a faucet that keeps running). In order to keep going, we find other solutions to keep up with the demand… now our bodies "steal", rob or borrow other hormones to help keep up with the workload (Pregnenolone). The other hormones are taken away from their daily job requirements to help the adrenal glands then the other hormones are all in distress. The domino effect begins. I was in constant "fight-or-flight" mode all day every day.

Required Lifestyle Changes for Adrenals:

- proper rest
- nutrition
- supplements
- removal of stressors

After lots of reading online articles, books, and seeking out consultations with functional practitioners, I had the various lab tests and blood work to determine why I am having so many odd symptoms. I did the lab test for cortisol (saliva test), gut test, food sensitivities, thyroid, vitamin deficiencies, and hormones test. I waited weeks for the results from my fasted blood work. One practitioner prescribed hormones replacement for the Whiley Protocol, and then others had supplements. My adrenal dysfunction not only compromised my adrenal gland production, but also caused hormone dysfunction, including hypothyroidism, insulin resistance, and estrogen levels. If your cortisol levels are low plus low DHEA and Pregnenolone levels are low, as well, then most all other hormones and body functions seem to be dysfunctioning and dysregulated, too.

My first few lab results showed:

- Cortisol and DHEA levels are low
- Liver detox system is off
- Thyroid levels are low
- Low hormones such as Estrogen
- Metabolic downregulation as my blood sugar irregular (cortisol controls blood sugar level) which means gaining fat

My symptoms were similar to what other athletes, like Christopher Kelly, (www.nourishbalancethrive.com) shared below on my podcast over the years:

- Bloated belly
- Brain fog
- Mild depression
- Dependency on coffee – caffeine
- Headaches if ate any sugar including fruit
- Chronic fatigue during the day and workouts
- Poor recovery from training sessions
- Difficulty sleeping then tired all day
- Low libido
- Allergies - stuffy nose all the time
- Light sensitivity

- Random injuries that took longer to heal
- Cold during the day - hands and feet
- Night sweats

My complaints/problems/symptoms:

- Poor sleep (trouble falling to sleep and waking up 1:00 a.m. – 3:00 a.m.)
- Weight gain and muscle loss even with clean eating (low carb/sugar) and exercise
- Blood sugar regulation problems
- Low energy levels
- Tired body and poor recovery from exercise
- High heart rates at low speeds/pace
- Muscle weakness
- Frequent headaches after eating (blood sugar problems)
- Emotional, frustrated, and tense
- More…

My Prescribed Supplements:

[The supplement list below includes what I took daily for a few months based on my lab results. **DO NOT go buy any of these supplements and just use this as another example until you get your specific functional lab tests conducted with a functional medical doctor or naturopath health coach.** The specialists will prescribe which supplements you should order from your practitioner and not buy at the local drug store, a wholesale warehouse, or grocery store.]

Talk to your practitioner before taking any supplements. This is my prescription for my imbalances and I over-supplemented myself since I over-researched for help.

This isn't for everyone as I am a special case with many issues, but just to give an example:

- Bone broth or collagen supplement to heal gut
- Detox protein shake in the morning (Dr. Sage created mix to help liver function)
- Oil of Oregano drops two times per day
- Red Ginseng drops
- Licorice Root drops
- Adrenal gland support
- Magnesium Calm drink mix
- Liquid Minerals
- Pregnenolone and DHEA (first month-drops)
- Fish Oils with Vitamin D (morning and evening)
- Blood sugar balance supplement (before meals)
- Neurotransmitter support (improve memory loss/brain fog)
- Branched Chain Amino Acids (BCAA)
- Vitamin C
- Glutamine (added in my protein drink) to help avoid muscles loss
- Vitamin B-12 drops
- Cod liver oil
- A-C Carbamide
- GI Revive
- Probiotic
- Multivitamin
- Orthomega
- GLA
- Pantothenic Acid
- Bioabpatogens
- Co-Enzyme Q-10
- Dopamine

- Protein powders and even some "Mr. Henry's" magic fiber cleanse
- Cortisol Manager in evening to help regulate my Cortisol (high cortisol levels 12:00 p.m. – 3:00 a.m. cause to have difficulty sleeping). Cortisol should be highest in the morning and lowest in the evening.

As you can see, an imbalance of your hormones cortisol and DHEA create chaos in multiple systems in your body. The supplements I took were suggested by plans, not just from one doctor, but a collection of recovery plans. Big mistake and not recommend. Again, I am sharing my crazy mixture of treatment plans to help you learn from my mistakes. Don't do what I did, especially without proper lab testing and professional guidance.

My Adrenal dysfunction Recovery Food Plan:

- Low carb, higher fat, moderate protein food plan (combine fat/protein/carb meals to provide steady energy release
- No coffee or alcohol
- Tea: liver detox tea and blood sugar balance tea in the day.
- Evening - digestion or calming sleep tea
- No sugar-> headaches -> increases blood sugar levels -> up insulin- fat storage.
- Avoid all fruit as it raises and drops blood sugar too quickly (combine with fat if needed)
- No gluten, commercial dairy, soy, corn, or peanuts (for sure no gluten) to help heal gut and digestion.
- Eat upon thirty minutes of waking (protein), eat every two to four hours to avoid low blood sugar (hypoglycemia)
- One to two tablespoons of coconut oil in the evening (mix with cinnamon)

My lifestyle changes in the first phase of recovery:

- DE-STRESS and LAUGH more. Chronic stress mode won't shut off so I have shallow breathing all day long (anxious, uptight)
- Easy walking nature walks without a cell phone or music. Focus on nasal breathing
- Yoga - ideally restorative, deep breathing
- Learn how to relax with deep breathing and mind-body exercises- create awareness all day
- Morning sunshine (ideally but at work.)
- Basic mobility - range of motion exercises (tissue mobility/lymph)
- Test Heart Rate Variability (HRV) to be over eighty. (SweetBeat)
- Sleep when dark: 9:00-10:00 p.m. bed and wake 6:00-7:00 a.m. (ideally, however, I am at work by 5:00 a.m. and to bed by 9:00 p.m., but now even at 8:00 p.m.)
- Use low-intensity exercise as relaxation, not for weight loss or performance gains
- Get more steps per day (movement), stress management and low-carb eating for weight loss
- Take a fifteen to twenty-minute nap in the afternoon when possible.
- Change work schedule - cut back on training group sessions and replace with admin time to catch up on work projects.

As I review my blogs from over the years regarding my health problems, I realize I probably was living in what some people call Stage Two adrenal dysfunction for five or more years before I really notice the obvious symptoms of Stage Three adrenal dysfunction – and hit the wall or rather hit the pavement when I stopped riding my bike that one Saturday, or when I was sick on the party bus. I missed all the red flags along the way until the big major ones that were impossible to ignore.

One red flag should have been when I was trying to get pregnant in my late thirties (I was a late bloomer in finding my perfect mate and "all in one" amazing husband). When I started going to the Seattle Reproductive Clinic and to a fertility specialist acupuncturist, nothing worked. My hormones were very low, follicle size too small, and my eggs were limited. I had signs of fertility issues, but the standard protocol was given to me, which was to take pills and shots to improve the levels.

I am sure the fertility clinicians probably were not familiar with HPA Axis dysfunction, adrenal dysfunction, and the domino effect it caused to the entire body systems including sex hormones. The clinic did my basic blood lab work a few times, weekly tests, hormone shots, and many ultrasounds to find the right time to create a baby. I was told my estrogen levels and other issues were low, but they didn't know how else to help me except to spend $20,000 on In Vitro Fertilization (IVF) treatments that only have a thirty percent (30%) chance of working at my age, which was thirty-five at the time.

As I look back over the years trying to get pregnant, going to the fertility clinic and seeing the fertility acupuncture specialists- my stress was probably the source of my fertility problems. At the same time, we were trying to get pregnant, my stress levels were probably always too high back (2008) as I owned my own small business fitness studio and over scheduled my entire days plus every weekend. If I knew now what I needed to know back then, I may have been able to heal my adrenals and hormone levels with the right treatment plan in order to get pregnant. However, I always believe everything happens for a reason, so I had to accept I was not able to get pregnant and there was a big reason for it somewhere. Neal and I had to become okay with not getting pregnant and creating a family together even thought we would have been amazing fun parents. I must have another mission and purpose in life other than being a mother to my own children. At least, that was what I told myself.

Over the years, I have done lab tests to determine what was off balance in my body. What did all of my multiple blood, pee, poop, and saliva lab tests tell me? My test results varied over time with treatment plans, lifestyle changes, and supplements but gradually the adrenals healed but something else was wrong. I still had/have a gut infection, a parasite, low white blood cell (sign of infection), and low thyroid plus other areas that need to continue to be supplemented (Omega 3, Vitamin D, and Iron).

As I learn more about nutrition and health in my educational programs, I believe almost everyone has some type of gut infection, parasite, or leaky gut wall lining, but are unaware of the problem because the symptoms become the norm for us. Please be aware that skin rashes, brain fog, gas, or a bloated belly are not normal, neither is running to the bathroom after eating. Those are more red flags we ignore every day.

Leaky gut symptoms, parasite, and fungal infections can show up in other areas of your health, according to the nutritional Therapy Association. If you have a parasite infection you have more symptoms to worry about and treat. A parasite by definition is "an organism that lives in or on another organism (its host) and benefits by deriving nutrients at the host's expense."

My many lab test results showed I had deficiencies in multiple areas. I am sharing my results as *an example* of why we need to get specific lab testing that most traditional medical doctors and insurance companies do not include.

Here is a sampling of what my functional labs showed at the time of the test:

- Adrenal dysfunction: Low cortisol (high or low is not ideal)
- Low DHEA and excessive Cortisol: DHEA ratio
- Low B12 vitamin deficiency and gene mutation in B12
- Leaky gut syndrome
- Low free testosterone, DHEA, and Pregnenolone
- Low Coq10 and Low vitamin D
- Low iron- anemic and Low thyroid
- Mediator Release Test: many food sensitivities detected
- Mitochondrial Krebs cycle dysfunction

Obviously, I was a walking over-supplemented, over-achiever, adrenal dysfunction, type-A personality, competitive athlete who was over-educating herself to recover/heal as fast as possible. I was never satisfied with one practitioner or doctor's protocol, so I continued to be on a mission to find the perfect healing solution. I wanted to be on the fast track program (adrenal dysfunction from living the fast-paced life). I was determined to get the right answer or, at least, wanted to hear a different solution.

Not only did I have prescribed supplements and hormone drops to take three times a day, I also added various herbal supplements I would read about online or in one of the many books I ordered, or from learning about it on a wellness podcast.

What I needed to do was to slow down, breathe, and let time heal the body.

One of my favorite practitioners in the Seattle area, Dr. Keesha Ewers, had me take the MRT test to find out my reactions to foods. Crazy... the first test showed my <u>red</u> list: do not eat black pepper, catfish, coffee, corn, ginger, Kamut, lamb, rye, and turkey. Then, the <u>yellow</u> list was even longer. I can do without Kamut and I don't eat lamb or like rye, but coffee, turkey, and black pepper were in most of my meals. Five months later, I took the test again to find out black pepper, paprika, and pistachio were the only ones listed on my red do not eat list and the yellow list was not as long, but had different foods. Possibly, my gut and digestive health were improving, but not totally recovered.

Dr. Keesha gave me the other lab tests as Dr. Kalish and Christopher Kelly but of course I like to get multiple opinions! I kept searching for a practitioner that worked with Ironman triathletes – as they could understand the mentality of a type-A personality and competitive endurance athlete but it doesn't matter... anyone experiencing similar symptoms as myself is living life as some type of race. Ironman or not, life stress adds up and even creates odd food sensitivities.

"The Mediator Release (MRT) is the key event that leads to every negative effect your patients suffer. What matters clinically is that mediator release, and thus an inflammatory response has occurred – not that a potential mechanism is elevated. This is the clinical value of MRT®. MRT® is a functional measurement of diet-induced sensitivity pathways. MRT® simplifies a highly complex reaction and translates that into the most usable clinical information you can get – quantifying the inflammatory response to foods and food-chemicals.

Not only does MRT® give insight into inflammation-provoking foods and food-chemicals, but more importantly MRT® identifies your patient's BEST foods – the foods that form the basis of their LEAP Eating Plan. MRT® is the foundation of fully addressing food sensitivities and achieving the maximum outcomes in the shortest period of time.

Source: http://tinyurl.com/NowLeap

Not only do you need to change the way you fuel, train, and perform to improve your gut health and reduce various types of stressors. You also have to identify foods that are causing a negative reaction in your body (stressor) even if they are otherwise healthy real foods such as black pepper, of all things. Make sure you talk to your trained practitioner to order the correct lab tests for your symptoms in order to get to the root cause, which is usually all a result of living life with excessive stress for an extended period of time. Too much of anything is toxic right?

I had lab tests from my various practitioners: Dr. Geoff Lecovin, Dr. Kalish, Dr. Keesha Ewers, Dr. Panah, Dr. Wheeler, Heather Glen and Christopher Kelly...plus I have continued to get lab testing through WellnessFX, as well as, my client's company www.arivale.com.

Here are more lab results from my retesting:

- Genova Diagnostics Organix comprehensive test (urine)
- Biohealth Laboratory Functional Adrenal Stress Profile – 201 (saliva) better, new urine test, I would suggest
- Biohealth Laboratory – GI Pathogen Screen with H. Pylori Antigen – 401H
- Blood Chemistry Functional Health Report – (blood lab test)

- US Bio-Tek Standard Food Panel test: IgG/IgE food sensitivity test

Throughout this healing time of my journey, I also tried colon hydrotherapy (not such a good experience or a pretty picture to paint) and then I discovered the benefits of healing from acupuncture and Chinese medicine. I even signed up for a three-month, expensive, and overpriced package from a local chiropractic that used spinal adjustments, decompression, and whole body vibration therapy to stimulate the spinal cord and cerebellum for healing the neurological-metabolic system. I didn't look at the costs. My health and well-being were worth it.

I look back at it all and think, I could have done additional walking, relaxation exercises, or slept longer instead of creating more stress by searching for the fast-track program. I was taking one step forward then two steps back. No wonder this health problem that was to take six to twelve months to heal from has taken over three years.

I went two times a week for three months for a neurological treatment by a local chiropractor believing it was the answer to my problems (good selling job on their part). I originally committed to their fancy gold package of six months, but quickly changed to their bronze package after I realized how much more money another treatment plan would cost. I continued on my quest to find the magic solution. I made appointments with two other well-known functional medicine doctors in the area to review all my lab tests (*huge* file folder by now) only to get the same response of which supplements to take as well as a multivitamin and an iron IV drip.

More money on the same thing...

I didn't worry about how much money I was spending, investing, or wasting on myself in order to be healed. I was searching for the quick fix and not more supplements. I don't want to even calculate the thousands of dollars I spent on my search for the speedy adrenal fix. Perhaps the answer was to do nothing and let nature takes it course, although I didn't trust that solution.

Next, I went to my traditional doctor for lab tests and help only to be given low thyroid medication. A hypothyroid is usually a symptom of other hormonal imbalances and medication isn't always the solution. I had gained so much weight in a two month time period; I thought I must have thyroid issues and metabolism problem, right? After taking the thyroid medication, the weight still didn't come off. I was devastated as I had small hopes that thyroid medication would solve everything. Of course, it didn't.

I continued to cry out for help knowing there was a problem with me. My endurance workouts were still horrible, my muscle strength was lost, I couldn't eat any sugar without getting an immediate headache, my sleep was irregular, my recovery from training took days, and I was fat. How could I not have something wrong with me? I kept looking for someone else to give me the answer I was seeking. I wanted to have my energy so I could train, race, and lose all of that uncomfortable annoying fat on my body.

I started to learn more about stress, gut infections, and parasites after listening to podcasts with Paul Chek. Not only did I agree with everything he discussed, but he shared stories in his "Eat, Move, and be Healthy" book that were just like my own. The insight and a different perspective I gained from his articles, books, podcasts, and videos led me to become a Holistic Lifestyle

Coach with the C.H.E.K Institute. The knowledge I gained from the C.H.E.K practitioners was a life changer: Health starts from the ground up and it is essential for all of us to integrate physical, emotional, mental, and spiritual parts of ourselves to create the WHOLE person from the inside out.

Overall well-being doesn't just consist of our exercise and nutrition program or taking lab tests to determine which supplements we need to take three times a day (yes, I had my "pill bag" with me for months), but we must learn our own *why* and *what*?

Why are we feeling the way we do today? How did we get here and where do we go from here? What is our roadmap?

As I continue to heal and repair from the inside out and work on the WHOLE me, I persevere to be more inspired to get educated as a C.H.E.K holistic life coach Level 2, Kalish Method Practitioner, and soon a Nutritional Therapy Practitioner (NTP). I am motivated and driven to brand The WHOLESTIC Method program and grow my *"The WHOLE Athlete"* podcast. I am on a mission to share information and educate others who may relate to my story.

Another reason to continue learning and sharing my knowledge via blogs, books, manuals, and podcasts are because of the amount of information out there that is confusing and misleading. What we read and hear isn't always correct. Remember, you can't believe everything you read on the internet, said Abraham Lincoln.

One can never learn enough, especially in the world of health and wellness and learning how to take charge of our health. Nowadays, I see my acupuncturist, Ying, whenever I feel off or out of balance or have an injury. The search for answers on healing, repairing, and health education never ends, but make your health a priority and improve the WHOLE you from the inside out.

The majority of my health problems are a symptom impacted more by burning out the adrenals since cortisol is required to regulate blood sugar levels. The point I am trying to make here is to improve your health from the inside out, you need to do some research to find the right functional doctor or lab to get the detailed testing as with WellnessFX, Nourish-Balance-Thrive, or a Kalish Method Practitioner.

Don't you want to know what is under your hood of the car?

The Attempt to Return to Racing

16

"Live out of your imagination, not your history."
- Stephen Covey

After six months of adrenal treatment, I felt I was ready to racing or at least participate in endurance events. In the fall of 2013, I began to slowly ramp up the mileage of my running as I was gradually feeling better inside and out.

First, I had to deal with being a spectator in the 2013 races I'd had to withdraw from due to my health issues. I was registered for Honu 70.3 and Ironman Canada in Whistler as you used to have to pre-register for races a year in advance. I had to learn how to be a spectator instead of being an active participant. This was an emotional experience for me. I had a new and completely different perspective of experiencing triathlon races which only increased my desire and motivation to return to the playing field as quickly as possible.

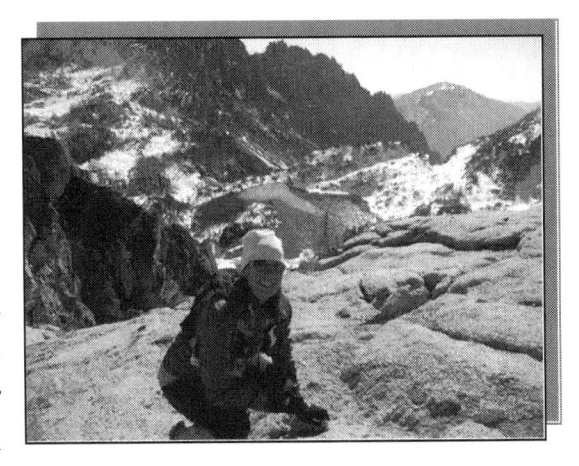

One of the emotional challenges for me in 2013 was watching Ironman Hawaii instead of competing in the World Championship. We had our trip to Kona reserved and paid for in advance before my adrenal crash and health problems. My goal was to qualify for Ironman Hawaii World Championships at Ironman Canada Whistler, but you know what happened to that plan. The vision board I'd created the previous year had the time goal of 10:15 magnet on my fridge to remind me daily of my Ironman goal finishing time and to qualifying time for Ironman Hawaii.

Eventually, I got to experience an endorphin high again, this time in the mountain air instead of in Kona running Ali'i Drive to the finish line. After we returned from watching Ironman Hawaii in Kona 2013, Neal and I joined our friend, Joel, to complete one of the most amazing and challenging twenty-two-mile hike/run in one day just outside Leavenworth, Washington called the Enchantments. This hike is one everyone must put on their bucket list.

The Enchantments are just that… enchanting and require not only hiking or running, but also bouldering and climbing up sides of a mountain (Assured Pass). One suggestion is to not go in late October as we were climbing up the mountain trails in snow and sheets of ice. It's not ideal conditions for a novice and triathlete road girl such as me. I was extremely terrified a few times and screamed frequently when climbing the ice wall. It is good to get out of your comfort zone and do something new every once in a while in order to grow and transform.

The beauty of the Enchantments mountain pass is so spectacular; one must stop many times and push the pause button.

Stop, look around, and breathe.

Be still and be present.

After we reached the peak of the pass, we started our descent. On the way down, we finally got out of the snow and ice packs and now we could do more trail running. Somehow, I was able to do a total of twenty-two miles that day with running back to our condo after the trail ended. I was so excited to be healed. I may have been too excited, but the hike gave me my confidence back that I could be athletic again. I needed to stop living life as a race.

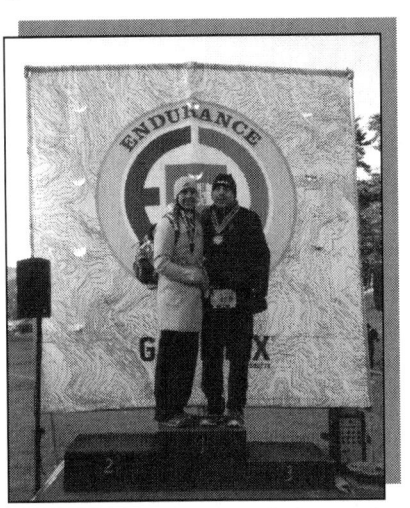

Since the Enchantments hike was successful for me, I decided not to withdraw from the other race/event we were registered to do in December 2013. Neal and I did one of our favorite annual events which were another beautiful trail hike/run. The North Face 50K trail run/hike in the San Francisco-Marin Headlands the first weekend of December was hilly, but with stunning views and smells of eucalyptus trees). I actually completed the 50K trail event, but mostly by hiking fast and running the flat (very few) sections as well as the descents. I was much slower than in past years, but I was able to finish the event with a smile on my face.

Again, another confidence booster that I was almost healed from my adrenal blowout. I thought I was ready to race triathlons again in 2014. I still had my base, aerobic foundation/engine, that I could hike, walk/run for hours without fatigue, and I was ready to rebuild my strength to make my comeback in Ironman Triathlons.

Not so fast.

Once again, I was searching for the fast track program; mind over matter.

The year didn't start out as planned to make my return to racing. On New Year's Day 2014, I was running a sandy trail in Palm Springs area when I pulled a muscle in my calf. The previous weeks, my running pace started to pick up and my strength was improving. Now, I'd had a new setback to my comeback. I had to do some acupuncture and body treatment to get the inflammation down but the injury was taking longer to heal than as expected. I had an MRI which revealed a small tear in my meniscus (padding-small cushion behind the knee).

No worries... I can heal up and return again to my training.

This was really a red flag from the Universe telling me I was doing too much and trying to return to endurance training too quickly.

Where was the pause button? I must have lost it again. I needed to stop and reassess my roadmap. Was I doing too much too soon? I wanted to believe I was magically healed in a six to twelve months recovery time.

When your body is off and the hormones are out of balance, healing from injuries takes much longer (red flag). I needed to find patience and slow down again, to stop with endurance training and focus on short workouts, mobility, and strength. Another setback meant someone was trying to tell me something.

Since I was regaining confidence in my recovery, I registered for Honu 70.3 in 2014 as my "A" race and then I would decide on registering for Ironman Canada Whistler if the 70.3 triathlon was a success. I forgot about the red flags again and pushed that darn pause button for the year.

Never ignore the red flags, messages from the Universe, or your gut instinct to rest more. Just two weeks before my flight to Kona, I went for a morning bike ride with a few clients who I'd never ridden with outside of the spin class I'd taught. The bike ride was to be my pre-race tempo and then I was going to go for a tempo run.

My plans rapidly changed.

About twenty minutes into this early Friday morning ride, I somehow got knocked off my bike, flew right over the handlebars, and smacked my head, knee, hip, ribs, and hand on the ground. 911 was alerted and on their way.

I was a bit broken and beat up, but my bike was okay. All cyclists worry about their bike over their body first. My helmet must have come off my head since I had a huge hematoma bruise on my face (beautiful look you can't hide well), banged up knees (so much for those bike pants), deep cut on my hip bone, and my ring finger was all bloody and painful. I ended up breaking a bone in my right hand, but the worst part was having my Tiffany's wedding rings cut off my left hand. I've never yelled so loud as when they were removing my rings. I thought they'd take my fingers, as well. I now take off my jewelry when riding my bike and I always wear gloves.

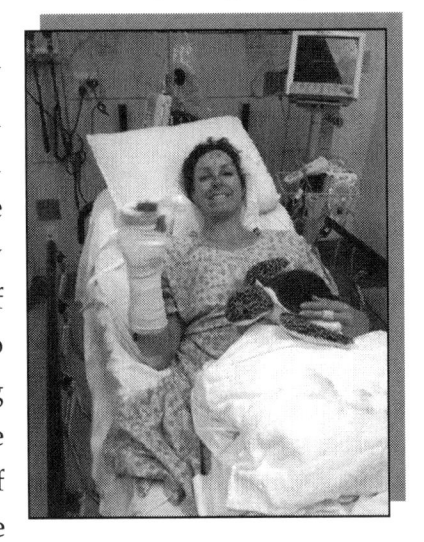

Not only did my wedding rings get cut apart to save my fingers, my hand had to be set in a cast. To make the situation even worse, the ER doctors set my broken hand bone in the cast incorrectly, which made me less than happy. I'd already had a hard cast (at least it was pink) on my hand and wrist for four weeks until they did an x-ray to check the healing only to find out it was not set right and out of alignment.

Everything happens for a reason, right? What was this reason now?

I could have a funny-looking disfigured pinky finger bone for the rest of my life or go to another hand surgeon to re-break the bone and reset it in a new cast. I ended up leaving the "Group Death" ER doctors to find a hand specialists surgeon as I was not going to have another set back again. That summer, I had to get yet another surgery to pin my hand bone back together correctly and set it with seven little pins. I'd already had shoulder surgery in 2006 from a bike crash (in the rain) and a foot fracture (probably related to my bunion) in 2009, so I was not as scared going into my third surgery related to my Ironman training.

Sadly, I discovered I had a new reputation of being accident prone and requiring surgeries, but I had to quickly remind clients and friends that the accidents or injuries were almost ten years apart so I am not as accident prone or cursed as people thought. How embarrassing. I am starting to seem like a careless rider and slightly becoming a klutz. *Or* is this an outcome of my lack of focus and trying to do too much at once in life and sports? The association of multi-tasking and Debbie go together. I am always trying to feel productive by doing too much, but I don't agree my bike crashes were a result of my carelessness or lack of focus.

Just to clarify my other bike accident was in 2004 when I fell off my bike on a rainy day going up to a sidewalk ramp. The back wheel must have slipped in the oily pavement. The accident created a small fracture in my forearm (brachioradialis) four weeks before my first Ironman Hawaii race. I raced anyway with only a month of indoor training and no swimming prior to race day in order to heal my fracture.

A year later, the same bike crash resulted in a shoulder injury that required surgery. Of course, it was right before Ironman Hawaii, so I had to watch the race in tears inside on the sidelines instead of physically racing in 2005. My surgery, scheduled the day after I arrived home in tears, depressed over not being able to race my second Ironman Hawaii race, to repair a large, torn labrum and a cyst in my left shoulder. Rehab from my first surgery started immediately.

In 2009, the morning after I returned from an amazing week girls/clients trip on a yacht in the Caribbean, I somehow fractured a bone in my foot on my morning run. I don't know why or how, but my foot started hurting during the run and I had to get back to my car. I ran/walked/hobbled for two miles. The next day, after getting an x-ray, I discovered I'd fractured my second metatarsal and needed surgery number two to get a plate and screws in my foot. The fracture was most likely a result of running with poor mechanics due to a bunion on my big toe.

Another setback for my 2014 return to Half Ironman and Ironman Triathlons was someone telling me I was doing too much too soon. I was forced to be sidelined again with a big hematoma and broken hand while watching yet another triathlon I was registered for. Not the best way to battle depression. I needed to find the positive in these experiences and discover what the learning opportunity was to be for me.

I flew to Hawaii with a cast on my arm, a hematoma on my forehead, Band-Aids all over and a smile. I used this as an opportunity to connect with the Island gods and healing lands of Hawaii. After all of my setbacks, I was forced to approach life with a positive attitude and find the opportunity or gem from each experience A positive mindset is required in life.

What was my plan of action?

My vision board needed to be recalibrated and perhaps not focused on racing again. Why don't I focus on improving other aspects of my life instead of finding happiness on my bike or in a race? Or why should I change?

What do I want to achieve in life?

Why do I train and race?

What makes me happy?

What do I want my legacy to be?

The summer of 2014 was the perfect time to dig deep on my *WHY* while healing my injuries from the bike crash. That accident was a major sign I wasn't ready to race yet. Since I had to have hand surgery in July, my return to my biking was prolonged again. I wasn't able to ride my bike from mid-May (when the bike crash occurred) until mid-August. I discovered how therapeutic my bike rides were for me during the months when I was not able to ride, especially in the summer weather. My bike and run workouts were my therapy times and my happy place.

After everything, I was finally able to compete in a small, fun, local, sprint triathlon in September 2014 and actually placed in my age group. The win was great for my confidence and happiness. But, was I ready to start training for races yet? My external injuries may have healed on the outside from the run accident in January and bike crash in May, but were my internal injuries healed up? Was there another red flag or obstacle going to arise out of nowhere? Another setback or rather life lesson to learn?

Over time, I was able to get back to training again, but my pace, power, and strength were a struggle. I was so much slower and heavier than in the past that my recovery time seemed to take weeks instead of days. Now, what was going on with my body and health? Was this ever going to end? Didn't I deserve to be healthy again from the inside out? I thought I was being patient, slowing down, pushing the pause button, and then resetting, but was I actually walking the talk?

Instead of trying to be patient in this healing process, I continued to test, becoming more annoyed and frustrated. Honestly, I just wanted to be as strong, fit, and lean as I was in the past. I thought it would make me happy and alive again. I need a new plan, a new vision, and a new approach. I needed to create a new roadmap to my healing program because what I had been doing the last year wasn't successful.

I reached out to my podcasting friend and Kalish Method practitioner, Christopher Kelly, to do more lab tests to see why I was struggling with strength, weight loss, and a slow recovery. After doing more lab tests, Christopher resolved to see what my root cause was. The results showed I still had a gut bacterial infection that was not healed since discovered in my first BioHealth lab test in April of 2013. The BioHealth GI pathogen screen test (401H test) involved doing a lovely four-day stool sample test (scooper into a small bottle). The first test and now re-test in 2015 still detected I had a "Blasto" parasite infection which showed concern for overgrowth of microorganisms in my gut. Wonderful!

The BioHealth lab results explain, "Parasite infections can be silent but destructive, perpetuating chronic stress on the infected individual 24/7 by raising cortisol levels and causing inflammation."

The BioHealth lab tests in 2013 and 2015 continued to find:

*"Escherichia coli. Conclusive evidence showed that bacteria called Escherichia coli are present in your stool culture. It is normal to have this type of flora in your intestines. However, the amount of Escherichia coli that is present may indicate a dysbiosis in the small or large intestine which is an **imbalance between the beneficial and harmful bacteria in the gut**. This imbalance may lead to **poor digestion, poor nutrient absorption and the overall rejection of some key nutrients which can have very negative effects on the body**, such as reduced immunity, increased infection or even infestation.*

Blastocystis hominis. *The stool antigen test results also indicate that you have a parasitic infection called **Blastocystis hominis**, commonly referred to as Blasto."*

Another roadblock to my recovery? Patience was needed... and is still required today. I had to stop and take a deep breath. I don't have cancer and I am not going to die. Life could be much worse. I'd had enough of these non-stop roadblocks, obstacles, and setbacks from reaching my goals. Perhaps the changes I'd made were not enough. Once again, I was frustrated, annoyed, and depressed, but who could I blame other than myself? This constant struggle in the healing and recovering process was exhausting. Why couldn't I get myself healthy from the inside out? What was my struggle? Why did I have this internal imbalance and chaos for so long?

But I don't have cancer and I am not going through chemo as other people are in my life. I am going to be okay... just a few sacrifices and changes in my lifestyle habits are required.

Earlier in my story, I shared that the healing process from

adrenal dysfunction is partially dependent on getting the right lab tests to find the correct supplements to heal the internal system. The other half of the healing treatment was reliant on me. In order to recover, I needed to continue working on me. Evidently, that was not happening enough as I still had parasites living inside of my gut. What an awful image. Paul Chek believes ninety percent (90%) of us have some type of parasite or fungal infection from the high sugar diet, stress, and other habits that create a susceptible environment to become infected.

You can learn more on parasite infections from Dr. Mary Meyers as she shared on a blog:

"Having a parasite can be a scary thought. However, you are not alone. Parasites are far more common than you think. It's a myth that parasites only exist in underdeveloped countries. In fact, the majority of the patients I see have a parasite. As you will see, parasites can cause a myriad of symptoms, only a few of which are actually digestive in nature.

<u>*What is a parasite?*</u>
A parasite is any organism that lives and feeds off of another organism. When I refer to intestinal parasites, I'm referring to tiny organisms, usually, worms that feed off of your nutrition. Because parasites come in so many different shapes and sizes, they can cause a very wide range of problems. Some consume your food, leaving you hungry after every meal and unable to gain weight. Others feed off of your red blood cells, causing anemia. Some lay eggs that can cause itching, irritability, and even insomnia. If you have tried countless approaches to heal your gut and relieve your symptoms without any success, a parasite could be the underlying cause for many of your unexplained and unresolved symptoms.

How do you get parasites?

There are a number of ways to contract a parasite. First, parasites can enter your body through contaminated food and water. Undercooked meat is a common place for parasites to hide, as well as contaminated water from underdeveloped countries, lakes, ponds, or creeks. Unclean or contaminated fruits and vegetables can also harbor parasites. Some parasites can even enter the body by traveling through the bottom of your foot.

Dr. Meyers' 10 Signs You May Have a Parasite
- *Unexplained constipation, diarrhea, gas, or other symptoms of IBS*
- *Traveled internationally and remember getting traveler's diarrhea while abroad*
- *History of food poisoning and 'your digestion has not been the same since'*
- *Trouble falling asleep or wake up multiple times during the night*
- *Skin irritation or unexplained rash, hives, rosacea, or eczema*
- *Grinding your teeth in your sleep*
- *Pain or aching in your muscles or joints*
- *Fatigue, exhaustion, depression, or frequent feeling of apathy*
- *Never feeling satisfied or full after your meals*
- *Diagnosis of iron-deficiency anemia*

The signs of a parasite can often appear unrelated and unexplained. As I mentioned previously, there are MANY different types of parasites we are exposed to in our environments. I typically see *parasites causing more constipation in patients than diarrhea, but some parasites are capable of changing the fluid balance in your gut and causing diarrhea. Trouble sleeping, skin irritations, mood changes, and muscle pain can all be caused by the toxins that parasites release into the bloodstream.*

Often times, these toxins cause anxiety, which can manifest itself in a different way. For instance, waking up in the middle of the night or grinding your teeth in your sleep are signs that your body is experiencing anxiety while you rest. When these toxins interact with your neurotransmitters or blood cells, they can cause mood swings or skin irritation. Parasites have a unique life cycle, where they can rotate between dormant and alive.

If you think you might have a parasite, I encourage you to find a functional medicine physician in your area so that they can order a comprehensive stool test for you. My motto is, it all starts in your gut, and your gut is the gateway to health. A healthy gut makes a healthy person.

Source: http://tinyurl.com/MeyersParasite

The keywords on my parasite test lab results included that the Blasto parasite infection: *"leads to poor digestion, poor nutrient absorption, and overall rejection of some key nutrients."* There was no surprise as to why I wasn't able to get my speed back in my legs, improve my performance, or shorten the recovery time from workouts. My friend, Blasto the Parasites, had been living in my gut for over two years and still today I fight this infection. Acupuncture two times a week is my current program to fight this Blasto infection.

I blame the water we swam in for the Las Vegas 70.3 World championships. Or, should I blame myself for accumulative stress that left me with a weak immune system?

You have to wonder why triathletes are permitted to swim in the water on a race day when swimming is not allowed the rest of the year. One needs to be concerned when swimming in water where you can't even see your own hand in front of your face and, even worse, when you come out of the water with brown coloring on your skin and suit. What parasites and other unmentionables were we swimming in?

That won't happen again for me. The visual of Blasto parasites hibernating in your body is not comforting and they are obviously difficult to kill off especially when they are hatching more eggs inside of you. My possible infection swimming in dirty water for a triathlon wasn't the main reason for my parasite as I was already stressed to lower my immune system to create an ideal home for these buggers.

Christopher Kelly helped me start a three-month program to kill off the Blasto parasite infection. Of course, I was always looking for additional solutions to speed up the process, so I also started seeing my Chinese medicine acupuncturist guru, Ying, again to assist in the Blasto murder. I wanted these Blasto parasites out of my system. I was blaming them for my health problems and the low thyroid.

I needed to find patience; the lesson to be learned again in this situation instead of feeling depressed and angry. What was the opportunity in *this* experience to grow and transform from now? I wanted to return to feeling fit, lean, strong, and happy I had to learn what makes me content and relaxed.

I had to reboot my healing program and repair my gut health. As you know by now, healing requires patience, discipline, and commitment which I obviously didn't always have except when training for races. The mindset I had in a race now needed to be put into my health treatment plan. Nutritionally, it was simple for me. I had a need to avoid gluten and sugars, but I was already used to that habit from the previous few years when I got into the low-carb living and metabolic efficiency. Now, I had to focus on being strict with my foods to heal my gut by eliminating any gluten, no sugar, add strong probiotics, and multiple gut healing supplements.

As of the writing of this book, it is time to re-test to find out if the "Blasto" parasites are gone, but I am hesitant to find the truth, as well as spend even more money for another test. Instead, I've ordered another three-month supply of the "Blasto Kill" supplements from Christopher's company www.nourishbalancethrive.com.

My running is gradually getting faster and stronger, but it is a long process. At least, I am injury and pain-free—knock on wood. Through all of this, I've discovered the need for *patience* and that darn pause button in order to not only rebuild my running strength, endurance, and speed, but my internal health. Every part of our body is connected, inside and out.

For me, it was never simply the adrenals or the thyroid or the Blasto parasite. I repeat this to myself, my new mantra is: slow down, push pause, and reset. Take deep breathes and create personal speed limits each day with speed bumps along the way. Inhale "slow"... exhale "down." Recovery means more rest, not easier workouts. It is all about balancing the nervous system. I needed to figure out how to stimulate my parasympathetic (rest and digest) nervous system much more frequently than my constant sympathetic nervous system. As people often say, "You can rest when you are dead."

Obviously, life should not about racing through each day in such a hurry and being addicted to busy-ness. Unless you are looking to shorten your life span

That was then... This is now   17

"The only person you are destined to become is the person you decide to be."
- Ralph Waldo Emerson

Let's dive into the major question...
How much is too much? When does too much become toxic and too little is a deficiency?

Less is more, but how much do we need to slow down to avoid crashing in life? Now, you probably understand more about me than I know myself. My goal now is to walk the walk and practice what I preach by continuing to work on slowing my pace and catching those red flags in advance in order to avoid another internal crash which I am still healing from a few of the various side effects (as my parasite infection and low thyroid).

It is so easy for me to revert back to my old habits and personality as they are tough to break. I am trying to avoid walking on the fine line of going back to my old ways. Even with all the red flags, setbacks, and roadblocks I have experienced over the past few years, I continue to focus on transforming into a new better version of myself. I keep up with my swimming, biking, and running workout sessions as if I was training for a race, only with a different mindset and personal rules.

Why do I continue to do triathlon training after all of my setbacks?

It's simple. My workouts are therapy sessions.

Also, it's because I love to exercise and the feel-good high from endorphins. I love swimming, biking, running, lifting, and more. Exercise is my career and my hobby. It's my routine, my passion, and my therapy time. I don't think training and racing need to be a negative aspect of our lives if we find happiness in it and not try to live each day as if it were a race.

What if we change our perspective on life, training, and racing by just pushing that pause button more frequently and resetting your life in all aspects? I find myself often needing to add longer transitions or breaks between my daily events in life as my major stressors are not my workouts, rather the speed or pace plus intensity I would approach the entire day. I actually have to stop and listen to what my body is telling me. If we are quiet long enough, we can get feedback from our body. Walk instead of run. Take a rest day with no exercise at all. Maybe that's the message. You see, my body knows me better than I do.

My approach to life, work, and training is slightly different as I learned from my many red flags what I was able to change and shift in my life. Over the last few years, in order to recover, heal, rebuild, and transform into a new and improved individual, it has required serious reflection on my lifestyle, work, nutrition, training, and the toxic people I'd allowed into my circle. I had to make necessary changes in my life, inside and out, in order to avoid going backward into that dark hole, I found myself in March 2013.

My new approach and mindset toward living my life has changed over the years based on my improved outlook and reflections. We have a choice how we want to live our life each day. Our attitude is everything. I try to soak up the *joie de vivre*, enjoyment of life and the laid back attitude—*c'est la vie*—you find in the French countryside, Italy, or Hawaii. My intense personality is gradually becoming more chill and I am working on not being as hard on myself. It's still a work in progress. Now,

I approach my afternoon solo workout sessions on my bike or a run as my time for mental clarity and to activate my creative brain while feeling calm and peaceful in the fresh air and in the outdoors. It is time for *me*, time to disconnect in order to connect with myself. No distractions with phone calls, emails, administrative work, or social media posts.

I focus on improving my lifestyle, work schedule, social life, relationships, and training habits to be more of a part of my own personalized version of The WHOLETSTIC Method journey.

What exactly did I change?

- ✓ Fun Fridays, for starters. I don't teach spin class anymore on Fridays at 5:30 a.m. Rather than filling the time with clients; I blocked the early morning time off for my workout date with my husband: lifting weights, running, or biking. Monday to Thursday, I start work at 5:30 a.m. with clients so Friday is now reserved for sleeping in or waking up without an alarm. For twenty years, I have had to work at 5:30 a.m. or 6 a.m. every weekday – so one weekday without an alarm is a treat.
- ✓ A new work-client training schedule. I switched my availability for appointments on Mondays, Wednesdays, and Fridays so I do not stay at my studio past 3:30 p.m. I block off two hours those days to work on my writing, study for my Nutrition Therapy Practitioner course (NTP), help out my WHOLESTIC Method online coaching clients, podcasting, and actually having dinner with my husband. Tuesdays and Thursdays, I work a double with clients from 5:30 a.m. – 11:00 a.m. and then again

from 3:00 p.m. to 7:00 p.m. I'm okay with not taking clients the other nights. We must set boundaries with our schedule to limit work hours and add more quality and focused time for family and friends and not always be available for text or emails.

- ✓ More sleep. I am now very serious about getting eight to nine hours of sleep each night. If I don't, I take a nap whenever possible in the afternoon when I feel sleepy so I don't feel exhausted. The nights I don't work late, I may be in bed around 7:30 p.m. or 8:00 p.m. by the latest to get my quality sleep.
- ✓ No alarm on the weekends. In the past, I was very strict in setting my alarm on the weekends to wake up in time for Saturday Masters Swim Workout at 7:00 a.m. and on Sundays for meeting friends or clients for a long run. These days, I don't set an alarm so I can wake up when my body tells me it is ready. If I don't wake up in time, then I obviously needed the extra rest.
- ✓ No scheduled group training commitments on the weekends. On the weekends, I stopped organizing any group long bike rides or group long runs. I go for a long bike ride after my swims with Neal when we are ready. No rush, expectations, or stress. I enjoy riding alone or else I feel stressed or anxious during my bike rides or feel the need to compete or race with others. Sometimes, I may be slower, feel stronger, or be faster. Solo workouts can be more rewarding and beneficial instead of pressure to perform at someone else's level or pace. It's better to go with the flow, Your body and mind will tell you what it needs.

- ✓ I am flexible about my training schedule. My swim workouts during the week are still with the Master's group at noon, but I don't stress if I am a few minutes late and I even get out early if I feel tired or mentally not into it. I have turned around in the parking lot at the club to go home for a quick rest break or nap when my body tells me it needs to slow down and reset.
- ✓ No garbage training in the "Black Hole." I listen to my body as to when to take an easy workout or a rest day as it ends up being a "garbage" workout anyways. Lesson learned here for sure. Why bother running when I can't move my legs very fast and they feel like dead weights? That is when a nice therapeutic walk in the beautiful outdoors with fresh air is much more beneficial than a slog.
- ✓ Solo afternoon weekday workouts. My bike days are based on the best weather days, but I still block out afternoons to ride year round as it is my mental therapy break from work - plus great brainstorming time. I listen to my body to decide what ride, or no ride, I am going to do that day, but also be flexible if I don't feel like riding.
- ✓ Red Flag Alert – pay attention to the signals. I head to my acupuncturist at any sign of fatigue, sluggishness, or health problems as he always knows what treatment to do. I trust his knowledge and the Chinese medicine philosophy to help me heal and treat injuries on the inside and out.

- ✓ Limit the coffee and caffeine. Instead of drinking too much Bullet Proof fat coffee each morning, I make my French press coffee with a splash of heavy cream or add a tablespoon of brain octane oil - Medium Chain Triglycerides. I try to drink more herbal teas and tonics during the day instead of caffeine, even though I love good coffee roasters.
- ✓ Eat right for my type. My body feels the best on a low-carb/high-fat diet. Eating more healthy fats and proteins keep me full and satisfied for hours. If I don't have time to pack food such as raw almonds, cashews, and/or walnuts with some raw goat or sheep cheese or an avocado when I am hungry during work, then I often add a nutrition protein shake with MCT oil for brain power. I stay full for the morning hours and I don't need my main meal until the afternoon.
- ✓ Practice what I preach. I continue to avoid processed foods, sugar, gluten, and grains most of the time. I follow the 80/20 rule – where you eat real food right for your metabolic type (more on this in The WHOLESTIC Method manual) eighty percent (80%) of the time and then, twenty percent (20%) of the time, you eat foods that are not ideal like a homemade thin crust organic pizza or a gelato in Italy. I keep on my food plan as often as possible, but sometimes have a "cheat" meal, especially if my husband, Chef Neal, prepares it for me or when traveling abroad. If I don't eat right for my body, I get a headache and/or stomach ache so I am more motivated to keep strict on my eating habits.

- ✓ Continue to retake lab testing. My supplements continue two to three times per day, but they change based on my current lab results which I continue to retest two to three times per year. I tend to be anemic and I'm still trying to kill "Mr. Blasto," my annoying stubborn Parasite infection. Typically, my lab tests show that I am low iron, b-metabolism, Glutathione, and branch chain amino acids. I take Probiotics, Fish Oil with Vitamin D, Iron, BCAA complex, Thyroid supplement, and Multi-Vitamin for athletes by EXOS Thorne. Sometimes, I take a month off of supplements as I don't think it is wise to depend too heavily on augmenting our diet, but rather eating the right foods instead to fulfill our needs.
- ✓ Commit to an evening ritual to unwind. I try to wind down and unplug from the day by heading to bed earlier to read a few pages in my book and write in my gratitude journal. I often play yoga or meditation music in our room (SONOS music system) with playlists off of Pandora music app.
- ✓ Go with the flow. My racing schedule is still a question as I don't feel ready to race at a competitive age group level for a 70.3 or full Ironman distance triathlon. I want to race 70.3 and even an Ironman if I am capable of placing first in my age group. I have raced enough to not need to finish a race just for the fun of it. Maybe this is the wrong mentality and it will change in a year. At this time, I continue to heal from the parasite infection in order to improve my health, blood work, and energy. I would like to compete in marathons and triathlons again if I won't be setting

back my progress and I am physically capable of performing my best. Plus, I can't help my competitive nature.
- ✓ Race less and travel more. Instead of spending so much money on racing each year, we started a travel fund. Neal and I plan on traveling somewhere around the world every two years. In 2014, we went to Italy for two weeks and the fall of 2016 we headed to Spain. The amount of money I have spent on race bikes, wheels, hotels, airfare, and registration fees, plus all the fueling and gear equals out to many trips to some amazing city around the world. We want to create our own bucket list and travel more. Besides, traveling with your spouse is wonderful for strengthening your relationship and creating memories together.
- ✓ Push and slow down as needed. The pause button. I don't jam-pack my schedule as much as I did in the past. I don't feel the need to rush from clients at my studio to my swim workout or meeting someone to bike then rush back to my next client. Pause. Slow down. Don't rush. I dislike being late to an appointment, so I need to continue being cautious when scheduling any appointment. Focus on no stress.
- ✓ More is not better. I have finally gained a "less is more" mindset. My approach to my triathlon training schedule has shifted as well as my daily life responsibilities, or at least I am working on it. Less is more. Honestly, this is a major challenge for me as I always want to do everything. I am finishing a book, a manual, and a workbook while I am starting an

intensive nine-month program to become a certified Nutrition Therapy Practitioner (NTP) while owning and operating my own private fitness studio.
- ✓ Build up more with fewer breakdowns. Anabolic vs. Catabolic training. Each week, I commit myself to three to thirty-minute strength training sessions in with metabolic blasts or HIIT training for at least one of the workouts at my studio with my clients or by myself, although with clients is always more fun and a more intense workout. More strength training is key for my health inside and out.
- ✓ Not to overschedule. Finding time for everything I want to do will always be a challenge while I own my own business. My body definitely needs yoga in my weekly schedule, but I can't figure out how to find more time for a yoga class for myself unless I take away time from my husband, sleeping, or swim practice. Instead, I teach more yoga for my clients as they keep asking me for more anyways. Teaching yoga is not nearly the same as practicing yoga, but it is better than no yoga. Discover the challenges or obstacles and find solutions.
- ✓ Take a "reset" break when the body calls for it. If you tend to be living life as a race each day. Relaxation time should be a daily priority. I listen to chill out, relaxation, yoga, or meditation music when at home doing chores or working on my computer as well as going to sleep at night.
- ✓ Clean out your closet and your relationships. Creating a toxic free environment at home and with friends. I had to terminate work relationships that caused more

daily stress than happiness. The weight was lifted off my shoulders after I made that major decision. Sometimes, you need to make major changes in your life in order to look out for yourself first. You may not notice how much stress and anxiety people in your life create until you step away from them. Take inventory and review your stressors and triggers.
- ✓ Create a time for yin and yang. Make sure we take care of ourselves with Zen time. This year, I started using essential oils for relaxation and healing with a diffusor as well as directly on my skin. I also would like to schedule massage/body treatment, foot reflexology and a facial quarterly. We like to work hard and train harder, but we need to make even more time for recovery.

My personal journey in transforming into a WHOLELISTC athlete continues as I wish to compete in another 70.3 Triathlon well as another Ironman someday, qualify for the Hawaii World Championships, and perhaps do one more New York City and Boston Marathon. I want to coach clients to become healthy from the inside out, which is why I'm getting certified as a Nutritional Therapy Practitioner (NTP). An NTP is a nutritional therapist who helps evaluate nutritional needs and makes recommendations for dietary changes. I want to help others restore their health by eating the right whole foods and nutrients, while they transform their lives and improve performance in daily life and sports. We are all unique individuals with specific genetic, ancestral, and geographical makeup.

What is your why and purpose in life?

Are you running from something or to something?

Why is it a struggle for us to stop moving and be still?

If we could all slow down and enjoy the journey, while eating real whole foods, maybe we would not have this increased rate of diseases and health issues in our country. Eliminate the quick grab and go coffee, scone and meals in a paper bag.

Life is not a race, so pace yourself each day. Make your life a journey with a few goals and objectives along the way.

Do you have a personal WHOLESTIC Method roadmap created yet?

Don't race away from something or someone in life. Take the time to stop and assess the situation, asking ourselves why are we doing what we are doing? What brings us happiness and joy? What robs us of energy? What is our *why* we have a choice how we want to live each day and we should not end our life with any regrets.

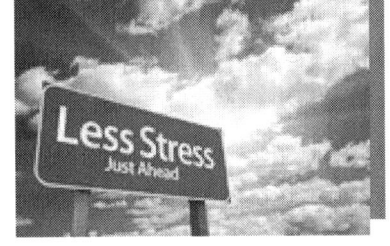

I begin another transformational stage in life just as a caterpillar turns into a butterfly each year. Each season I seem to learn something new about myself as I am pausing more often and listening to my signals.

What are you doing to improve the whole you and to transform each year as I plan to in my lifetime? Let's make a promise to continue to grow from every experience and set new goals in our annual The WHOLESTIC Method workbook roadmap, as we learn from experience.

We don't have to strive to act as Wonder Woman or Superman to live a long, healthy, and happy life.

Which road are you going to take?

Perhaps the road less traveled?

Debbie Potts

The Butterfly Transformation into the WHOLE Person   18

"When she transformed into a butterfly, the caterpillars spoke not of her beauty, but of her weirdness. They wanted her to change back into what she always had been. But, she had wings."
— Dean Jackson

As I transform into a new better version of myself, I also set up a newly-revised roadmap for myself creating, living, branding, and educating The WHOLESTIC Method philosophy. My new mission is to help others from going through what I have experienced the past five years.

I want to teach what I have learned from my past lifestyle habits and mindset to be successful. I believe everything happens for a reason, so I was encouraged to write this book and share my personal story to help others. From my journey, I now feel I have been given a new purpose in life.

My experience and journey can help athletes of all levels from the weekend warrior to the competitive top age group Ironman athlete to avoid this internal meltdown. It doesn't matter if you do endurance events; we're all susceptible to getting sucked up into the vortex of society's expectations to be busy, overscheduled and overcommitted in life.

You can avoid the internal health imbalances of leaky gut infections, parasites, adrenal dysfunction, and hormone dysregulation that lead to fatigue, depression, and weight gain.

Just stop, reset and reevaluate your roadmap in life, and then find the new road to transforming the whole you from the inside out with The WHOLESTIC Method.

When you focus on eating real food, exercising appropriately, getting quality sleep, reducing red flags and stressors, moving each hour, being kind to your gut and drinking more water, finding happiness in your life every day. You will become healthy on the inside and outside.

The additional benefits of improving the WHOLE you are slowing the aging process down in life and reducing the risk for now common health diseases. Based on my own health experiences, I know we cannot reach our peak performance and optimal health exclusively by long hours of exercise or following a low-calorie, low-fat fad diet.

It doesn't matter if you are a competitive athlete, a top executive, or a stay-at-home mom; we all need to focus on improving our WHOLE selves from the inside out. We all seem to struggle with letting go from society, so afraid we'll miss out on any experience, post, or comment.

I challenge you to take off those multiple notifications you have on your cell phones and computers. We can wait to respond to the email that just arrived in your inbox, the text message that flashed across your screen, or any of the other updates and notification alerts that will be there when we are ready to be *present* and *focus* on doing one thing.

Let's stop the multi-tasking and trying to do too much in one day. Let it go people. Tomorrow is a new day.

We have a choice in how we live our life each day and the schedules we create. If we could all stop trying to do too much in one day and prioritize instead of being an unfocused multi-tasker striving to finish in first place each day. We can stop striving to be an over-achiever and put quality over quantity. Habits are tough to break and create new habits in their wake, but it is possible. I am working on my new habits constantly and plan on not returning to my past way of operating in daily life. We all can maximize our performance in work life, personal life, and endurance sports by working on the WHOLE picture of health.

Chasing the Dream   19

"Twenty years from now you will be more disappointed by the things you didn't do than by the ones you did do. So throw off the bowlines. Sail away from the safe harbor. Catch the trade winds in your sails. Explore. Dream. Discover."
- Mark Twain

We need to own our goals or dreams that we set out to achieve in life without the pressure or influence of other peers.

As we go into The WHOLESTIC Method workbook and program, you will be asked to do some self-reflection, evaluating your lifestyle, habits, health, and discovering what makes you happy. We can all benefit from discovering and establishing what gives us a sense of purpose and mission in life. How do we want our "dash" to be written? The dash is the mark between the date we were born and the date we die. What's in between those dates is in our control.

In order to improve our WHOLE health, we need to block off some quiet personal time in order to go deep when creating our own version of The WHOLESTIC Method roadmap. What are you passionate about in life that makes you smile, laugh, and feel proud to be who you are? Why are we doing to dig into these questions you ask?

I find that in order to reduce the chronic stress we have been accustomed on thriving on each day, we need to step away, push that pause button I keep talking about, and reflect on who do we want to become?

Paul Chek taught us in our holistic lifestyle coaching program that we actually have three choices when we establish and recognize our goals or dreams:

1. Optimal: your decision is good for everyone and everything involved in your dream.
2. Suboptimal: your decision is good for you but not so good for everyone and everything around you.
3. Do nothing: not being present – instead of being indifferent.

Every now and then, we need to step back and reflect on who we are instead of reacting without awareness. The dreams or goals we set to help guide us get to the person we want to become (less stressful, anxious, and uptight perhaps) are influenced by two forces that work together to create balance... yin and yang. We need both in life in order to find the balance in our dream person we want to be that we love and appreciate.

If we find the right path and follow the journey that is going to take us toward making that dream a reality, then we will discover real joy, vitality, well-being, and love. Instead, we often end up making suboptimal decisions over time that lead to creating fear, fatigue, and depression in our lives. If we ignore all of the red flags that are presenting on the race course of life, then over time we now know what will happen to our health: fatigue, disease, and indifference toward life takes over.

How do you want to live life?

I know I want to find that happy fun Debbie who was racing her bike in Ironman Canada in 2012 cheering for every participant by their first name with a smile on her face, glowing with sheer joy in doing what she loved to do: ride her bike.

The C.H.E.K Institute philosophy, or Paul Chek specifically, teaches his students in the C.H.E.K Holistic Lifestyle Coach certification courses, about the "4 Doctors" you will ever need and express the qualities of yin and yang energy:

1. Dr. Quiet - "Chief Physician," sleep, meditation; if tired and fatigued then get more quiet time, spiritual development and anabolic rebound. Yin balance.
2. Dr. Diet - you are what you eat; what you eat and drink, the building blocks for the body, water-hydration - seventy percent (70%) of your body eats good food for a good body, metabolic typing, and satiation. Yin balance.
3. Dr. Movement - flexibility, warmth, functionality, moving the body, working in and working out. Stressing the tissues and pump blood through the body. Relax and contract the muscles. Yang balance.
4. Dr. Happiness - living code of conduct; who you want to become; what makes you happy, emotional intelligence, mental self - management. Identify what creates happiness in your life.

We have discusses the various types of stress in our lives which comes from physical, emotional, mental, and spiritual sources. All types of stress add up and must be in balance especially before planning a life, diet or exercise plan. What is the right path for you to continue following in life? We need to identify which areas we need improvement or more attention and which part is out of alignment: our soul, body, mind, and/or spirit?

The secret of working in is not to raise the heart rate; just move slowly and stay relaxed. Try deep breathing squat movement right after a meal to help digestion. Move nutrition and waste through the body, helps the breathing and movement through the body.

Excessive stress hormones or rather break down hormones (catabolic) are activated when we overstimulate the sympathetic nervous system then we suppress the parasympathetic nervous system. It is just like a teeter-totter, we don't want too much of the breaking down the body and not enough of repairing the body. When the sympathetic nervous system is turned "on" then the parasympathetic system is turned off. Perhaps this makes more sense of what happens when we have too much stress in our life. Those excessive stress hormones: financial, relationships, food, toxic environment, negative attitude, and exercise. Too much or too little. We need to find the middle of the road to drive down to continue our new journey.

Train hard, but rest harder. Athletes, remember endurance training is catabolic exercise, so we for sure need to add in strength training sessions to build up muscles (anabolic) as well as yoga or mobility exercises to help recovery. From time to time, it is more important and effective for performance if we take a nap or a walk instead of forcing a hard workout session.

Maybe you are not getting enough exercise because you are sitting at the desk, in a meeting, or in your car all day, then you need to carve out more time for workouts and movement.

If we want to perform our best in sport and life, we need to add more anabolic exercise and more time working in.

To Pace or to Race in Life? 20

"Sometimes the best thing you can do is not think, not wonder, not imagine, and not obsess. Just breathe, and have faith that everything will work out for the best."
- Unknown

I've already shared my new mindset toward my lifestyle, work, social, and training habits. What can you do?

I talked in the beginning of my story about how we are too connected to what is around us and too disconnected from our own selves. We are not able to focus while we train or perform in life each day because we are too distracted and scattered mentally. We need to get our mind right in order to reduce stress in our lives and find more inner peace. How do we get more connected to our own self? Seems simple, yet so challenging.

Let's begin learning how to reconnect with our feet to the ground and how to move correctly with baby steps.

A few of my tips to reduce chronic stress:
1. Focus on doing one thing at a time. Make a list and work on completing one item on your list before moving to the next one. Maybe set a timer for how long you are going to work on one project or task.
2. Learn how to connect your mind and your body. Try doing a squat, lunge or balancing on one leg to find the movement pattern that engages your glutes, your booty. How do your hips move? Where are your feet? Can you cork screw them into the ground and feel

that you are tearing the floor open with your feet? What does your upper body do when you squat? Observe how your hips, knees, and feet track in the mirror. What muscles do you feel working?

3. Disconnect every evening and most weekends. Try setting your alarm in the evening instead of only the mornings to disconnect. Set the time when you are to get off (turn off) your computer, social media, electronics, and television an hour before bedtime Limit when you read and respond to emails. Set a specific time in your schedule to respond to emails and when you are accessible especially in the evenings and weekends.

4. Stabilize your blood sugar levels and avoid overeating. Set rules up if you overeat or rather mindless eating after your last meal/dinner time. Set rules up that the kitchen is "closed" to stop eating after 8:00 p.m. or up to two hours before bed. Also, don't consume any sugar, alcohol, or caffeine in the evening that will cause the blood sugar to be unstable or to rise and crash.

5. Find happiness and make connection time. Keep a journal by your bed and write in it each night before bedtime. Include at least three things you're grateful for that day and why.

6. Manage and monitor your stress levels: test your heart rate variability each morning for five minutes using the Sweetbeat Life app. Take this time to do breathing and meditation exercises. Use your HRV numbers to help determine if you need to take a rest

day, easy workout day or reschedule a workout session.
7. Schedule time to be with people who make you laugh and smile. Just the opposite – cut out those relationships that drain you and that are toxic.
8. Make time for yourself and make a "deposit" for yourself each day or week. Perhaps this is going for a solo walk or bike ride or getting a manicure. Do something for yourself each morning to start your day with a smile on your face and a positive attitude to tackle the day with ease. Schedule massages, facials, or acupuncture.
9. Try to do something new once a month or even per quarter. When is the last time you did tourist activities in your hometown? Pretend you have house guests and take yourself out instead.

Here is what some of my peers and mentors suggested for their tips to reduce chronic stress:

"I know it is cliché but I love my meditation time. Twenty minutes is more than enough for me. When I start to feel overwhelmed by my ever-growing "to do" list, I take some time and do some breathing. Usually, I breathe in for six heartbeats in, hold for six, six, and six out, and six rest. And, just keep going until I feel better (or I fall asleep) or until twenty minutes is up.

I am also a big fan of strict working hours and strict email hours. For instance, I rarely check my email after 8:00 p.m. and that really helps protect my bedtime ritual. I like to pretend I am back at my government job in 2000 when I couldn't actually check my work email from anywhere but my cubicle even if I had wanted to. How awesome was that?

This is a trick I actually learned from you, Debbie. I fall back on WTF (What's The Focus) all the time. It's easy to feel stressed out if you have lost your focus (broadly philosophically speaking or specifically on a single task) but when you are sincerely engaged in only one focus at a time, you are the master of that moment.

Giving myself permission to indulge occasionally without beating myself up. Whether that be staying up too late watching Netflix, having a beer, skipping a working, eating the bun that came with my burger because I forgot to say "no bun, please" or choosing to not say "no bun, please" I remind myself that I am not as bad as my last bad decision anymore (or less) than I am as good as my last good decision. It's a continuum and as long as my lifetime average is skewing heavily to the "good side" that is all I owe myself.

And, finally: making up songs, doing terrible dances, dropping my pants, and letting my inner creepy clown out. I am not just talking about that patent phrase "incorporate play into your life." I am talking about sheer childishness. One of my favorites stress relievers is to see how shockingly juvenile I can rewrite the lyrics to the song that is currently playing. It's amazing how rude you can make Adele sound. I believe this is the reason why 'heart' rhymes with 'fart.'"

Brock Armstrong
www.skywalkerfitness.ca

"One of the best stress reducers is sleep. Getting enough sleep is critical for reducing stress. And personally, I think the guidelines that are out there are very conservative, meaning if you are under a lot of stress you will likely need a lot more than the 7-8 hours per night that you read about if it's going to have a significant impact on reducing stress. And once you start to get more sleep, it may take a year or longer to really start to get a deep recovery if you are in adrenal dysfunction. You will feel better fairly quickly, but the deep energy reserves can take a lot of long nights of sleep and many naps.

Exercise aerobically in a natural setting. This means to move your body without pushing it and do it outside, on a trail, in the ocean, up to a mountain, in a park, by a river. Exercising aerobically for bouts of even fifteen to twenty minutes if done outside can dramatically help reduce stress hormones and keep them lowered for a longer period of time than if you did the same amount of exercise indoors. The key here also is the aerobic part. That means low to moderate exercising heart rates. Setting a PR or pushing your effort to a maximum level will increase your stress levels, even if you feel like you got something good out of it. Those workouts should be done sparingly. (That's two tips in one: exercise aerobically and exercise outdoors.)

Be in the community. Alone time is essential for reflecting, but being with other people who are supportive and health minded will also help reduce stress. There's nothing like being with friends and laughing to help reduce stress levels.

Be spiritual. This will mean different things to different people. But basically it's a call to step out of your day-to-day and slow down, take a breath, reflect, connect with nature, which is the part of the world that will go on regardless of how you deal with stress. Experience that grandeur, and then feel how good you feel from it. Meditate. Be of service to someone you care about. Be of service to someone you don't even know. Once a day, think of one thing you are grateful for. My teacher, Brant Secunda, always says if you are alive you have at least one thing to be grateful for."

Mark Allen
www.markallencoaching.com
www.fitsoul-fitbody.com
www.art-of-competition.com

Tips from my C.H.E.K practitioner mentor, Jator Pierre:

1. Grow a practice of paying attention to the moments in your life that bring up emotional charge. Ask yourself what does this situation represent to me? How old do I feel emotionally? What might be underneath my initial story? Maybe said differently, we are never emotionally charged about what we think we are charged about. Allow yourself to have feelings; all of your feelings are beautiful, let yourself feel.
2. Play, play, play. Non-completive play. Let your inner child out, act silly, enjoy imagination, enjoy not knowing, can you connect with the imagination you had when you were three years old? When is the last time you played?
3. Invite more pleasure into your life, touch, massage, embrace, make love, dance, laugh, connect, and allow yourself pleasure. Engage in an activity daily that brings you pleasure.
4. Spend some time barefoot on the earth, even more, stress relieving get some unprotected sun at the same time. Time in nature or even simply gazing at a natural environment is something most of us miss at a physiological level and science is showing it is just as if not more important than nutrition.
5. Spend time in a community with similar values as yours, a community where you feel safe, secure, and understood.

Jator Pierre
http://www.wehlc.com

Ben Greenfield suggests a more simple approach… "Number one: learn how to say no. Numbers four through five: See number one."

Ben Greenfield
https://greenfieldfitnesssystems.com

I have discovered that the training isn't the stressful part or red flag alert for me as my training is my relaxation "zen" time for me. My high expectation to perform my best and my desire to be a certain fitness level as well as strength/power created added stress for me. I create that stress and I have control over it.

I have always been strong on the hills, so when people pass me (yes, I am competitive), I now find myself getting frustrated and disappointed in myself. Now that I am more aware of my "red flags" and triggers for stress, in order to avoid returning to adrenal dysfunction, I prefer to do most of my long bike rides and long runs solo so I don't get upset if I am slower than others or not as strong.

Here are some lessons I've gained as every experience is an opportunity to learn something new and to grow as an individual:

- Let go of your ego
- Be patient
- Be flexible
- You can't control everything
- Go with the flow
- Check in with your attitude- be positive
- Everything happens for a reason
- Find the lesson to be learned and grow from each
- Reassess and recommit

Epilogue
The WHOLE Transformation Ongoing Process

"The best day of your life is the one on which you decide your life is your own. No apologies or excuses. No one to lean on, rely on or blame. The gift is yours- it is an amazing journey- and you alone are responsible for the quality of it. This is the day your life really begins."
- Bob Moawad

I share my journey of living life as a race every day to help you prevent the internal and external healthy breakdown I experienced. Instead, I want you to join me in learning how to live each day as a journey.

If we could all learn how to be present, focused, and more connected in what we are doing this moment rather than multi-tasking through life. We need to give ourselves permission to pause, reset, and recalibrate instead of feeling guilty about focusing on ourselves before others especially family members.

Living life as a race doesn't end well. Stop glorifying the act of being busy and start celebrating being present and resetting. We don't need to master how to be over productive and over achievers. Stop and learn that it's okay to sit down and rest in between meetings, appointments, duties, and training sessions. We don't need to go non-stop from the time the alarm goes off in the morning until we hit the sheets at night. We can master the art of being still, quiet, and mellow to learn how to work in as much as we work out. Rest and digest instead of running from a lion each day.

You might surprise yourself to discover that your performance in daily life activities, duties, and athletic events improves when you institute the changes you've learned in this book. Know how to recognize those red flags and stressor alerts and stop feeling guilty if you are not busy or on the go twenty-four/seven.

We will improve our fat loss, health, and performance from the inside out when we work on treating the body as a WHOLE person with The WHOLESTIC Method. I am sure you will also improve performance in life and sports by stopping to push pause and reset as I am discovering as I transform into a beautiful, new butterfly.

Keep in mind that more is not better. Sometimes less is more. We need to find the delicate balance between the art of doing too much in life and doing too little. The more we do, the more risk for creating toxicity. However, if we do little, then we risk the chance of creating deficiencies in our lives. Make sure you are being more mindful and putting more deposits into your "wellness" bank account. Find that delicate balance between doing too much and doing too little.

Let's do this together. Join my journey to gain peak performance in life and sports while we stay healthy on the inside and out. Trust me, slowing down, not rushing, being present and focusing is an ongoing challenge for me, but it is gradually improving. You can improve, as well, and learn how to start living in the present and in the moment.

Life is not a race. Pace yourself. Find the right road and enjoy the journey along the way. Sometimes you just need to pause, reassess, and recommit to your plan. Make the appropriate adjustments along the way in order to be successful, but first, you need to create your personal The WHOLESTIC Method roadmap plan and define success to you, as well as your purpose and discover your *Why* in life.

The real trip to recovering from adrenal dysfunction is not all about lab tests and supplements. The real secret to recovery comes from deep within you and how you learn how to listen to your body and live life from the inside out. It is the lifestyle changes and mindset toward how we pace ourselves in our daily life is the key to healing from adrenal fatigue. It's how we show up in life and how we react and respond to all situations and experiences. Avoid getting sucked up into society's pressure that more is better.

Let's embrace change and avoid the addiction to busyness. Don't stop transforming into a new better version of you- be patient, believe in yourself, be grateful and continue your personal quest for eternal happiness. Heck, you just need to laugh more each day and be silly in order to live life to the fullest.

You have one life, so make it the best one.

Thank you for joining me in this new quest, living life as a journey and not as a race.

In good health,

Debbie Potts

About the Author

Debbie Potts is the owner, trainer, and coach of a unique personal training and group training boutique private fitness studio in downtown Bellevue, Washington. She has been in the fitness industry for twenty-five years and has continued to learn even more.

Her Fitness Forward Studio offers amazing total body efficient workouts using a variety of tools (or toys!) including free weights, TRX, Rip Trainers, sandbags, kettle bells, medicine balls, slam balls, wall balls and more plus we Pilates mat, yoga, functional strength movements, and sport specific exercises into our workouts.

Debbie's specialties include personal, semi-private and group personal training, mobility training, functional strength training, TRX suspension training, STOTT Pilates, Yoga, Rehab training, Metabolic Testing, C.H.E.K Holistic Lifestyle coaching, and USAT Triathlon coaching. Her next certification is to become a Nutritional Therapy Practitioner. She focuses on coaching clients with The WHOLESTIC Method while training clients on proper form, alignment and muscle recruitment. Debbie continues to educate her clients the skills how to listen, tune in and focus on their bodies during exercises for the best results - and to avoid injuries. Debbie believes in coaching clients to improve performance for life and sports with her The WHOLESTIC Method. Her coaching programs help clients focus not only on their exercise but also their nutrition, sleep, stress, digestion, hydration, movement, and happiness.

Debbie Potts

Debbie has been a competitive athlete for most of her life. She has been a top age-group triathlete and runner as well as a fifteen times Ironman finisher, five times Ironman Hawaii World Championship qualifier, and multiple Boston Marathon qualifier. Debbie completed over twenty plus marathons and half marathons. She coaches clients individually on metabolic efficiency, running, trail running, cycling, and triathlon events.

Check out her race results here:
http://www.athlinks.com/athletes/41680626/Profile

> **Get Connected with Debbie**
>
> **Text BURNFAT to 77094 to receive free tips and tricks on how to become a fat-burning machine.**

Find Debbie on Facebook, Instagram, Pinterest, and YouTube for more tips and tricks how to become a WHOLESTIC Athlete by working from the inside out to perform your best in life and sports.

Website: www.debbiepotts.net
Podcast: www.thewholeathletepodcast.com
Facebook: www.facebook.com/fitnessforwardbellevue
Twitter: twitter.com/thewholeathlete
Pinterest: www.pinterest.com/WholesticMethod/
Instagram: www.instagram.com/thewholesticathlete/
YouTube: http://tinyurl.com/DebbieYouTubeList
or https://www.youtube.com/user/FitForwardBellevue

Subscribe to Debbie's podcast, The WHOLE Athlete:

http://tinyurl.com/WholeAthleteiTunes or
http://thewholeathletepodcast.com

Learn more about Debbie's The WHOLESTIC Method coaching:

www.thewholesticmethod.com

Debbie's Practitioners and Peers:

http://kalishwellness.com/
http://www.nourishbalancethrive.com/
http://www.fernlifecenter.com/
http://drgeofflecovin.com/
http://www.chronicconditioncenters.com/exceptional-life-wellness-.html
http://www.sagemed.co/
http://sweetwaterhrv.com/
https://philmaffetone.com/
https://bengreenfieldfitness.com/
http://www.wehlc.com
http://chekinstitute.com/
http://nutritionaltherapy.com/
http://www.markallencoaching.com/
www.skywalkerfitness.ca/
http://bradkearns.com/

Debbie Potts

#lifeisnotarace
#lifeisajourney
#stoptheglorificationofbusy
#thewholesticmethod
#focus
#bepatient

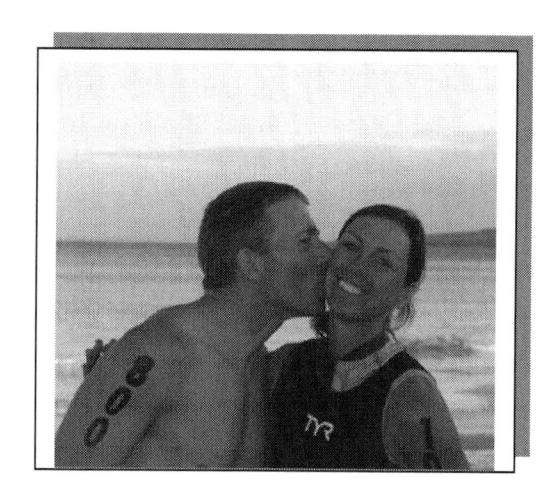

Made in the USA
San Bernardino, CA
29 November 2016